T0271534

The Diabetes Weight-Loss Plan

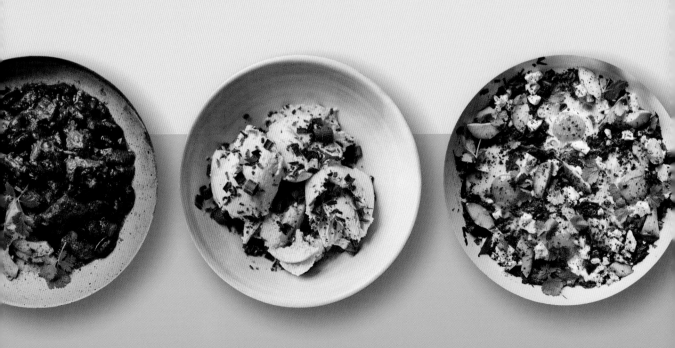

The Diabetes Weight-Loss Plan

Katie Caldesi

Kyle Books

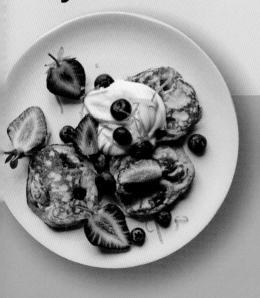
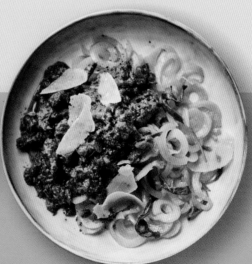
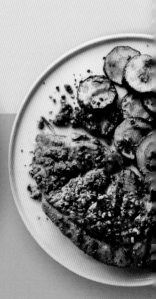

An Hachette UK Company
www.hachette.co.uk

First published in Great Britain in 2024 by Kyle Books, an imprint of Octopus
Publishing Group Limited, Carmelite House, 50 Victoria Embankment,
London, EC4Y 0DZ

ISBN: 978 1 91423 961 8

Distributed in the US by Hachette Book Group, 1290 Avenue of the Americas,
4th and 5th Floors, New York, NY 10104

Distributed in Canada by Canadian Manda Group, 664 Annette St., Toronto,
Ontario, Canada M6S 2C8

Publisher: Joanna Copestick
Editor: Isabel Jessop
Design: Paul Palmer-Edwards
Photographer: Maja Smend
Food Stylist: Lizzie Harris
Prop Stylist: Sarah Birks
Production: Katherine Hockley

A Cataloguing in Publication record for this title is available from the
British Library.

Printed and bound in China.

CONTENTS

Foreword

Giancarlo Caldesi

I was born in Tuscany, Italy, but have lived in England since I was 22 years old. I am a chef-patron, run two Italian restaurants, and, with my wife Katie, run a low-carb cookery school. I have recovered from type 2 diabetes and this is my story.

In 1998, I remember going to the seaside and realizing the water was so cold it hurt my feet; they felt like I was treading on glass. I should have known something was wrong then, but it was years until I did anything about it.

In 2009 I was working all hours at our restaurants; I would come home after a shift and devour the contents of the fruit bowl or cook a huge amount of pasta and eat it straight from the pan, as I was so hungry. While driving I would eat raisins, and at each garage stop, I bought chocolate or biscuits. But I still didn't realize anything was wrong with me medically.

My weight gain worsened, particularly around my waist, and I drank bottles of water to quench my constant thirst. I stopped playing football with the boys because my feet hurt so much. I developed gout and arthritis.

One day in 2011, I was driving home when my eyesight became blurred; it was really frightening, and it made me go straight to the doctor. Within days I was told I had type 2 diabetes. My HbA1c, a measure of blood sugar, was 49mmol/mol; the normal range is up to 42, and the pre-diabetes range is between 42 and 47.

I had textbook symptoms of type 2 diabetes: the weight around my waist; my constant thirst; the gout and arthritis. I was also always 'hangry' and spent every moment I could on the sofa, snoring. Both Katie and I went to see a dietician who advised me to cut portion sizes and reduce my sugar intake, and told Katie that her waist measurement meant she was in danger of becoming pre-diabetic. Looking back, neither of us took it as seriously as we should have done.

By 2013 I had worsened: my HbA1c rose to 79mmol/mol. In a bid to feel better, I gave up gluten. This meant I had to give up my favourite fresh pasta, the pastries I loved, bread, pizza and more. However I saw massive improvements within days. We were eating more vegetables, eggs, meat and fish and less 'beige' food. I had already reduced my sugar intake, too, so we were going low carb without even realizing! To confirm if I was gluten-intolerant, we saw nutritionist Jenny Phillips. Her tests revealed that I reacted very badly to gluten and she advised me to be scrupulous in banning it from my diet for good.

By 2015 I had lost nearly 3 stone and turned my type 2 diabetes into pre-diabetes, with my HbA1c now at 45mmol/mol. Both of us felt better, and over time we discovered that there was a whole world of low-carb eating.

In 2016 I was finally in remission from type 2 diabetes, with a HbA1c of 40. We met Dr David Unwin and Dr Jen Unwin who have helped hundreds of people put their diabetes into

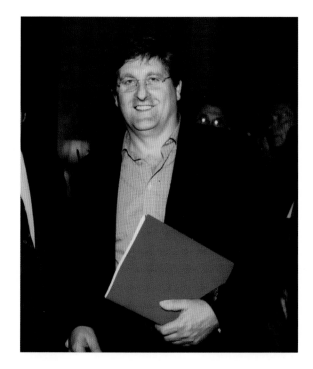

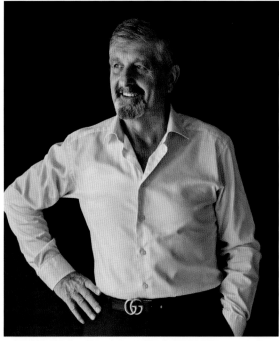

remission. Together with Jenny we decided to write our first book in this series, *The Diabetes Weight-loss Cookbook*. This led to a further 5 books about low-carb eating to promote weight loss and conquer type 2 diabetes. I feel I was really lucky to have had great people around me to advise me, and I still have. Support from your friends and loved ones can make all the difference.

My tips for maintaining remission

You need perseverance, determination and planning. Having a plan is so important to keep you on the straight and narrow; it gives you focus and makes you think, *Why should I deviate and feel terrible again?*

Be strong and develop a mental state in which you can overcome the cravings for carbs and sugar. It's most important that you disregard your brain wanting something sweet or starchy; your body does not want or need it. As you mentally adjust, you will become happy without sugar. By giving up sugar completely for 3 weeks, you will really notice the sweetness of everyday foods such as milk instead. The cravings for sweets, sugar, cake, rice and bread will pass. Now that I understand how my body works, I am more comfortable with disregarding cravings. Not eating the biscuit or going without bread for a week is very good, so congratulate yourself when you have made a step forward.

People ask me, 'What can we eat?' I always tell them that there are loads of good foods that you can cook or eat in restaurants. Whenever possible, choose whole, unprocessed foods and look at the creative ways given in this book to replace high-carb ingredients with low-carb alternatives.

On our low-carb courses, I find that people don't want to go out of their comfort zones, but I tell them their comfort zones are killing them! Please don't be obstinate. Dr Unwin told us that just six hours of high glucose levels can damage your arteries. If that's not motivation, what is?

I often wear a blood glucose monitor to keep an eye on my glucose spikes, as I know I am a sugar addict and I can go off the rails easily. I can't have anything tempting in the house. I had to clear out the cupboards and get rid of the 'mind-bending' junk food like biscuits and sweets. Even dates, raisins and jars of honey have to be on the highest shelf at the back, as I know I'll be tempted and I don't want to go back to feeling ill and being overweight. I like my new self and want to stay this way. So be honest with yourself, too – who are the chocolate buttons for – the kids? They moved out two years ago!

I do have a treat once a week – one of our low-carb desserts – otherwise I would feel too restricted. You could make some of Katie's chocolate muffins on page 184 and freeze them. When you want a dessert, defrost one in advance, that way you can't eat them all in one go. If I can do it as an Italian chef surrounded by pasta and delicious food, you can do it too.

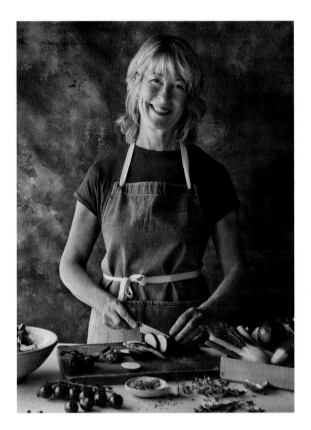

I'll highlight the questions that baffled me; I hope it helps you plan your own low-carb journey to health.

Dear Reader,

This is a letter we would like to have been sent when Giancarlo was first diagnosed with type 2 diabetes. We didn't understand the condition, how serious it could be, why he had it, or what we could do to help. With no medical or nutritional training, we found it hard to get our heads around it; we know how that feels. We needed to completely rethink everything we thought we knew about having low-fat food and plenty of carbohydrates.

As Giancarlo said in his foreword, we were lucky to find a great team to patiently explain blood glucose levels to us over and over again until the penny dropped. Our books are here to share that information with you. Be patient with yourself as you learn to understand type 2 diabetes. Read the science in this book, the pages on How to Start (see pages 10–17), the Meal Plans on pages 44–47 and the information, recipes and tips on our site www.thegoodkitchentable.com. Then fill in your own meal plan to follow. It is very important if you are on medication to speak to your health practitioner first and tell them you are following a low-carb diet.

I feel strongly that you should understand what happens in your body when you eat different foods. If we had known that, Giancarlo would never have suffered as he did. Armed with this knowledge you can fight against pre-diabetes, obesity and type 2 diabetes and restore your metabolic health.

Since Giancarlo's HbA1c levels have dropped to within the normal range, and his diabetes is in remission, life has been so much better; we didn't realize how ill he was before. Giancarlo feels great and I have a new slim husband who is full of energy and fun once more. It's been a difficult journey, but Giancarlo feels that if he can do it, then you can too. It's never too late to make a start.

The low-carb lifestyle is about eating fresh, natural foods that don't overload your bloodstream with glucose from sugar and starch. I'm passionate about helping people who read our books and take our cookery classes to prepare their own wholesome, nourishing meals rather than relying on ultra-processed foods. These changes are easy and don't have to be expensive. Let me show you.

Once you have your plan, get shopping, chopping and cooking, and enjoy it. Enlist help from family and friends. Make quick meals for two and family meals for feasts or batch cook and freeze; just stick to your plan. And if you go astray for a night, just get right back on your plan the next day.

I hope that the recipes will inspire you to put on your apron and take charge of your own health, starting in your kitchen. This book is the first step to your new life.

Your wellness is in your hands!

You can do this! *Katie.*

HOW TO START

Follow these steps to start your low-carb eating plan and enjoy the benefits of improving your metabolic health:

Read the science, more than once if necessary, and understand how your body works.

Look at the CarbScale on page 38 and decide your upper limit of carbs.

Count carbs – Read food labels and look at our carb swaps (see page 15), Dr Unwin's teaspoon charts (see page 20) and the recipes to compare the carbs in familiar foods and our recipes; it's fascinating. Calculate the whole meal, not just one portion; that's the nibbles beforehand, the sides, any dessert and what you drink with it. Jenny gives advice on how to do this if you aren't following a recipe from this book (see page 42). Keep noting down your carbs until it becomes second nature. After a while, you will naturally pick low-carb choices and you won't need to count anymore.

Look at the Low-carb Meal Planner on page 42 for ideas for basing your meals around protein, non-starchy vegetables and healthy fats.

Avoid ultra-processed foods and treats.

Ban the beige and eat a rainbow. Recognise carby foods easily: they are mainly beige. Resist them and replace them with colourful nutritious foods instead, see page 25.

Love your veg. Replace starchy carbs whenever possible with green vegetables. Above-the-ground ones like cabbage, courgette and salad veg are less starchy than below-the-ground ones like potato.

Give up added sugar in tea, coffee and sweet fizzy drinks. Eat low-sugar fruits such as berries and whole apples or pears rather than sweet fruits such as bananas, grapes and raisins.

Plan the week. Look at your diary and plan your meals. Copy the meal plan on page 204 and fill in the blanks. What are you going to have for dinner tonight? And tomorrow. Cancel the delivery app on your phone. Think at least two days ahead to avoid a 5pm panic and an ultra-processed delivery meal because you are craving carbs.

Start with three meals per day with no snacks, with a minimum of 5 hours between. You will not keel over! The whole point of losing weight is to release the calories stored as fat. Eating low carb allows your body to do this by training it to become a fat burner rather than a fat storer.

Weigh yourself twice a week. Monday and Friday mornings, to isolate the weekend. Do not attach emotion – it is just information!

Enjoy cooking! I know that is easy for me to say, as it is my passion, but I have watched so many customers at our school enjoy cooking, even when they thought they wouldn't! Get the family involved, even from a young age, and watch the workload disappear. Everyone can have a job.

Keep an eye on cost. Don't overbuy food: If you are likely to be out a couple of nights or you have

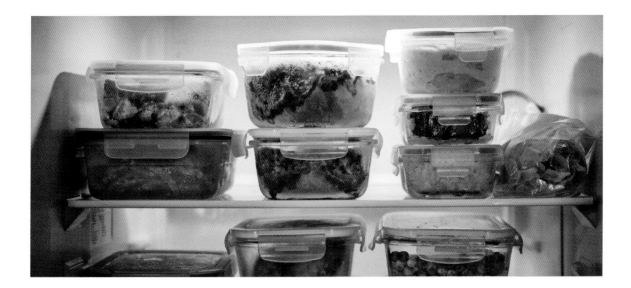

food you really should use up, don't buy too much. Look out for cheaper cuts of meat to use in the Simple Beef Stew recipe on page 114, frozen fish or chicken in the Quick & Easy chapter (see pages 76–111) or canned fish in Curried Fishcakes on page 93 or the Spicy Mackerel Pâté on page 80.

Batch and freeze. This chapter (see pages 112–129) is devoted to getting organized! Think ahead and cook just once a week to provide up to eight meals, each of which can be adapted; for example, the stew can be transformed into a lasagne, ragu, curry or chilli. I love it when I think I have nothing to eat and I look in the freezer to see my work; delicious meals ready to defrost and reheat in minutes.

Embrace your leftovers, and follow the principles of a 'continuous kitchen'. When I was a child, our leftover Sunday roast would be made into another meal on Monday, part of a sandwich for Tuesday lunch and so forth. The bones would be made into stock and we would finally finish the original roast as a soup with any leftover meat in it. And

that was without a freezer and a microwave; now we have no excuses. By cooking a large beef stew on a Sunday, you can freeze the leftovers in two portions, turn one into chilli con carne, and eat another as ragu.

Get saucy. To make up a vinaigrette, a spicy chilli sauce and maybe a chermoula, see the chapter on pages 62–75. These will keep in the refrigerator for a week or more and with the addition of soft-boiled eggs, a piece of fish or a chicken breast you can make quick and delicious meals in minutes.

High-days and holidays. Look at the Feast Days chapter (see pages 130–153) to see plenty of ideas as to how to celebrate while keeping low carb.

Remind yourself of your motivation. It might be serious; when Giancarlo turned 65, it made him think of his life ahead – or it could be trivial; I had a photo of me in a swimsuit on my refrigerator door for a while. I was happy with my figure when the photo was taken and looking at it encouraged me not to open the refrigerator door!

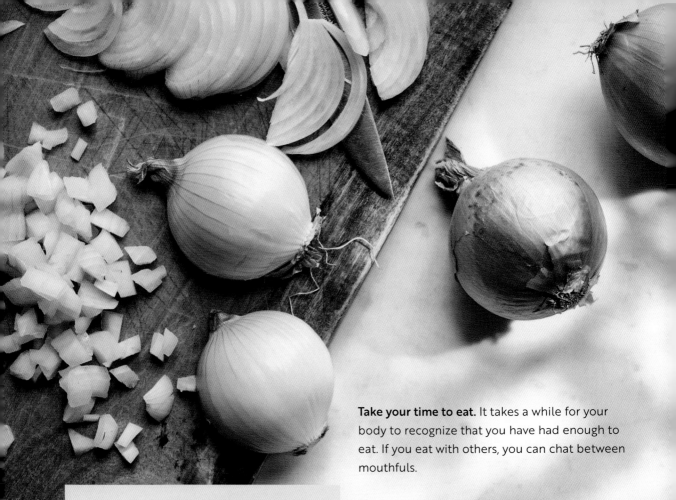

A few notes on temps, measures and sizes

Eggs can be any size unless specified.

What is a pinch of salt? My pinch is generous, around 3g (⅛oz), to give flavour. Reduce this if you have been told to by your doctor.

The numbers in the nutritional analysis of my recipes are only a guide, but it's accurate enough to tell you what is likely to give you a glucose spike.

What is the difference between a chopped and sliced onion? The photo on this page shows you – at the top is sliced, below is chopped.

Take your time to eat. It takes a while for your body to recognize that you have had enough to eat. If you eat with others, you can chat between mouthfuls.

Start your meal with fibre. In Mediterranean countries such as France, Italy, Greece and Turkey it is traditional to start a meal with a salad, antipasti or mezze; these take the edge off your hunger so you don't then devour a huge main course. And eating fibre before carbs lowers the resulting spike of glucose. Check out the work of Jessie Inchauspé, 'the Glucose Goddess', for more.

Acknowledge your comfort foods. There are plenty of healthy comfort foods in this book. Mine is toast, butter and Marmite with a cup of Earl Grey tea – not so bad, you might think, but I have seen the spike I get from a slice of toasted sourdough – not great. So now I love our low-carb bread that I can toast and enjoy.

Be prepared for travelling

On the way to a wedding recently, we stopped at a service station. Everything around us was made from sugar or starch. The few salads contained carbs, too. Giancarlo and my son Giorgio, who were wearing blood sugar monitors, ate rice-based dishes. When my other son Flavio arrived later, he saw the spikes on their monitors, so we ordered a bucket of fried chicken and peeled away the coating! On the way back from the wedding, we prepared for the same stop with our own low-carb picnic – and guess what? No spikes!

Move more

Use every excuse to move; sitting down is unhealthy. Incorporating physical activity into your daily routine is so important for reducing obesity and managing pre-diabetes and type 2 diabetes. Exercise helps lower blood sugar levels, it improves insulin sensitivity and it promotes overall well-being and energy levels. Get outside into the great big green therapy room, called 'outdoors'! Enjoy your endorphins, however you get them, from a brisk walk to HIIT, from cycling to swimming or dancing around your kitchen.

What to drink

Drink water: but that doesn't have to be boring. Try adding a couple of rosemary sprigs to a jug of water and leaving them to infuse for the day. Alternatively, adding washed strawberry hulls or slices of peach to water makes it delicious. And after straining out the fruit, you can fizz the water in a soda maker. Even better!

Can I have a glass of wine?

My friends know how much I enjoy a glass of wine, but as Giancarlo has to control his sugar habit, I have to control my wine o'clock craving. It's surprising to learn how many units of alcohol and calories there are in a glass of wine. Red or dry white wine are low in carbs so aren't off the menu, but this doesn't mean you can drink them limitlessly.

While moderate alcohol intake has been associated with certain health benefits, excessive or chronic alcohol consumption can have detrimental effects on the body. Choose alternative activities to relax: go for a walk, take a bath, read that book you have been meaning to start or phone an old friend. You'll still get the feel-good factor, and you'll feel better the next day.

Children and healthy eating

I have been asked on many occasions how people can get their kids to eat healthy food and not demand chicken shapes and chips. This is a massive subject and not one I can cover in detail in this book, but in principle, none of us, whatever age, should be eating junk food. Our kids were 10 and 12 and both had tummy fat, like us, when we changed the way we ate. I quietly removed the crisps, sweets, biscuits, cereals, fruit juice and ultra-processed foods and replaced them with nuts, small pieces of cheese, apples and tomatoes. I reheated leftovers for breakfast instead of offering them cereal and gave them whole yoghurt with vanilla extract and low-sugar fruits. I added small portions of pasta, potatoes and rice to our low-carb meals and they naturally lost weight without any mention of the word 'diet'. They are in their twenties now, eating moderately low carb, fit and healthy.

High-carb foods

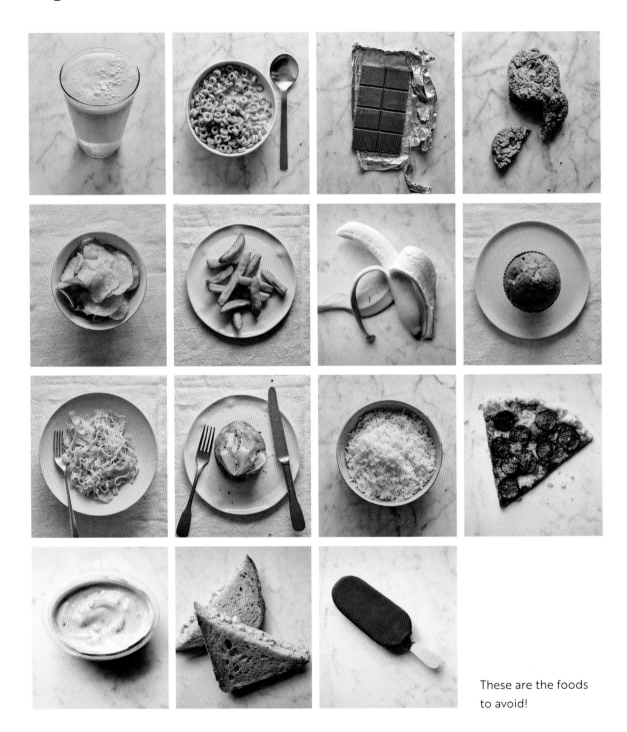

These are the foods
to avoid!

Low-carb swaps

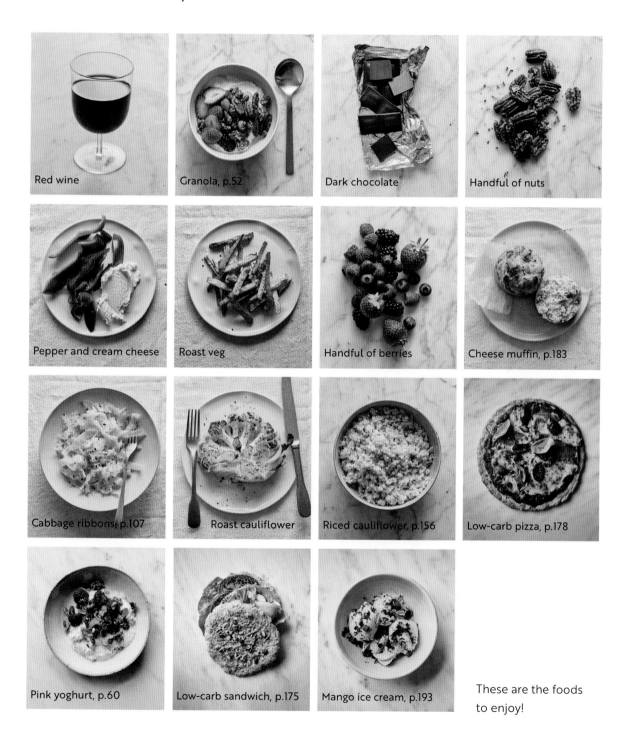

Red wine

Granola, p.52

Dark chocolate

Handful of nuts

Pepper and cream cheese

Roast veg

Handful of berries

Cheese muffin, p.183

Cabbage ribbons, p.107

Roast cauliflower

Riced cauliflower, p.156

Low-carb pizza, p.178

Pink yoghurt, p.60

Low-carb sandwich, p.175

Mango ice cream, p.193

These are the foods
to enjoy!

What to eat in restaurants

Since we run restaurants, we know how tempting it can be to overdo it at a dinner out. We have introduced a symbol, 'LC', for the low-carb options on our menus. Here are some helpful tips to enjoy a lunch or a night out without falling off the wagon.

Choice of restaurant – Have a look at the menus and choose a restaurant that will offer you a suitable choice. A pizza restaurant will have less choice than a steak restaurant but the latter may not be your preference or within the budget. Have a look before you go, so you know what you can order, and stick to it.

What to choose – You should be looking to eat an adequate amount of protein and non-starchy vegetables so you aren't hungry. This is not necessarily about eating less; it's about eating better. You need to be like Sherlock Holmes, looking for the sugar content, and don't go anywhere near dessert unless it is low-carb fruit or cheese.

Bread – Refuse the basket, however artisan or tempting it looks. Say yes to olives instead.

Wine – Tell yourself how many glasses of wine you are going to have and stick to it, enjoying sparkling water in between. I am not always good, but I try to stick to two: one at the beginning of the evening with olives and antipasti (so not on an empty stomach) and one later with the main course. I ask for a big glass of sparkling water with lime or lemon. Avoid beer and sweet cocktails (see page 132 for more on alcohol).

Sides – Ask to swap starchy carbs such as mashed potato, rice or chips to non-starchy vegetables such as sautéed spinach, roasted vegetables, green vegetables and salad.

Salad as the main course can be lower in carbs than a whole pizza, for example, but look out for sugary dressings and ask for olive oil, salt and pepper instead. If you can, get a few lemon wedges to squeeze over, which will be much better than a balsamic glaze or honey or syrup dressings. If possible, ask the restaurant not to add potato or grains to the salad and instead to have more leaves.

Starters plus a side might be better than a starter and a main – mozzarella, burrata, bresaola, beef carpaccio, egg-based dishes, spicy prawns, olives, sautéed mushrooms and rocket and Parmesan salads are all good options.

Main courses – Steak, chicken and fish without sugary sauces are all fine.

BURGERS

Have the meat, cheese and salad but ask them not to give you the bun.

CURRY NIGHT

Order vegetable sides instead of rice. Go easy on the dhal and chickpeas; they're better than rice but still starchy. Dry tandoor-cooked meat and fish are better than dishes with oily sauces.

CHINESE

Go for dry food rather than sugary sauces, such as roasted fish with ginger and garlic. Avoid battered food, and choose green vegetables rather than rice.

VIETNAMESE AND THAI

These can offer brilliant choices, with protein- and non-starchy vegetable-based salads and prawns – just say no to the rice, even if it's included.

MEXICAN

Avoid the nachos, rice and beans and go for meat or fish, Padrón peppers, guacamole and salad. Tequila shots are better than sugary cocktails and beer.

SUSHI AND JAPANESE

No white rice; instead go for sashimi, vegetables, salad and fish mains, but avoid sugary sauces. Choose dry sake over beer.

FRIED CHICKEN

Avoid it. There is almost nothing here for you when you are enjoying a low-carb lifestyle, though I have on occasion peeled away the coating and eaten just the chicken.

COFFEE SHOPS

The demand for low-carb food is getting stronger and bigger – in 2017 Starbucks introduced their 'Egg Bites'. Avoid ordering a latte (think of the milk sugar) and any syrups.

THE LOW-CARB LIFESTYLE

Helping to bring back the joy of general practice

Dr David Unwin, GP

Back in 2012 – like so many GPs today – I found myself exhausted and demoralized. If someone told me I was about to start a wonderful new clinical service that would have worldwide influence, I would have been quite astonished!

And yet that is exactly what my psychologist wife, Dr Jen Unwin, and I did at the Norwood GP surgery near Liverpool, England. As a consequence, ten years later we have appeared on TV and radio, written 40 articles for journals and newspapers, and spoken at conferences all over the world, and our work has been translated into 18 languages! The basis of all this interest is that 50 per cent of all our patients with type 2 diabetes who have 'cut the carbs' have put their diabetes into drug-free remission (that's 129 people so far). They no longer need expensive medications, so each year we save the NHS about £65,000 from our diabetes drug budget. Imagine the savings if every GP surgery in the UK was doing this! In fact when we published our data in 2023[1] 97 per cent of all our patients who were interested in improving their type 2 diabetes had actually done so, and had maintained that improvement for 30 months! The good news didn't stop there. We had also achieved significant improvements in all our measures of cardiovascular risk: things like weight, blood pressure and blood fats. We are part of a growing international body of opinion who feel that improving diet is key to improving the nation's health. If you are reading this book, perhaps you agree. As you will learn, the

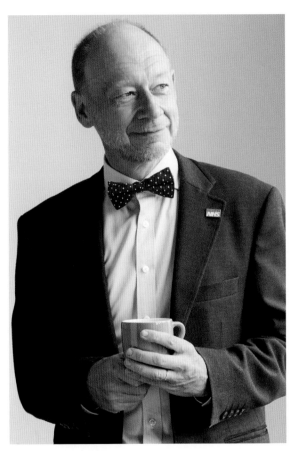

guiding principles of our work are surprisingly simple: just avoid the sugary and starchy foods that put your blood sugar up.

The magic is how to replace these staples with delicious meals, so you actually enjoy the process of improving your metabolic health. It is key that this is a lifestyle, not a diet.

How did this transformation come about?

Like all practices, we had seen an exponential growth in the prevalence of obesity and type 2 diabetes – an epidemic that has occurred across the world. Managing diabetes and its complications puts a huge strain on our clinics. Here in the UK we now spend £1 billion a year on the drugs for type 2 diabetes and its tragic consequences. When I was a new GP in 1986, we had just 57 cases of type 2 diabetes; by 2012 this had increased eight-fold to about 470. It's odd that I never thought about why this epidemic was occurring.

I remember my advice at the time was fairly standard

- Everything in moderation
- Eat a little and often
- A high-fibre breakfast is important
- Move more
- A low-fat diet is preferable

Over many years this advice seemed to make little difference. I became frustrated that patients were clearly ignoring my advice and concluded, like many doctors, that changing diet didn't make much impact, it was better to just start the medication early. You see, it was easier to blame the patients rather than my own advice, and yet that was the common denominator! No matter how many medications I prescribed for my patients with diabetes and obesity, many of them didn't seem to experience significantly better health. The whole thing was just so depressing. As a young doctor I had been so keen to make a difference, but by the age of 55 I felt as if I had failed. (I probably should say a word in defence of medications here. Yes, I still offer them, just more carefully and after sharing both the pros and cons with the patient concerned.)

One patient changed everything

Then one day in 2012 a patient with diabetes changed everything. I had asked her to come and see me because she had not been ordering her diabetes medication for some time. I planned to explain how foolish she was, but I was in for a shock. She had lost so much weight and, oddly, her blood sugars were normal, even after many months without medication. In a horrible turn, she was not just cross with me, she was furious, even wondering if I was properly qualified. She explained, 'Even a schoolboy knows that starchy carbs like bread, cereals and rice digest down into a lot of sugar, so they are a poor choice for someone hoping to reduce blood sugar.' She suggested it was better to eat a low-carbohydrate diet with more green veg, meat, fish, eggs and full-fat dairy: all low-carb foods that don't put up blood sugar nearly so much as carbohydrates. Apparently, over a decade of diabetes treatment, I had never mentioned this to her. She discovered the low-carb approach online and the results astonished her – and me. She felt I had a lot to learn, and it turned out she was right. Up until that day, I saw type 2 diabetes as a chronic, deteriorating condition, one that over time would inevitably need more lifelong medication. In 2012 I had *never* seen a single case of drug-free type 2 diabetes remission. Now in 2023, I meet proud, amazing people in every clinic who have done just that. My 'heartsink patients' have become my heroes! This case is similar to Giancarlo's and so many others around the world: people who don't accept that having type 2 diabetes means an inevitable decline.

Choosing your diet may be part of choosing your future

Thinking about this eight-fold increase in the prevalence of type 2 diabetes, it's not possible such a phenomenon can be due to genetic change in just a few decades. My experience supports the idea that the whole problem is environmental, not genetic. I believe it's just a matter of changing our food environment. I simply don't accept the situation as hopeless, and we have the data to prove it!

Part of all this is the rise and rise of 'junk' or ultra-processed foods. In the UK these 'food-like' substances now make up 56 per cent of all the calories in the British diet[2]. According to the BBC, the three most common problems are: industrialized bread, pre-packaged meals and breakfast cereals. This book is all about helping you to make delicious, healthy food instead of relying on those packets and pre-prepared supermarket foods.

Teaspoons of sugar

Dietary carbohydrates are the main drivers of blood sugar and so are problematic for people with type 2 diabetes. But this is complicated, as various dietary carbs affect blood glucose differently. Table sugar itself is easy to understand,

FOOD ITEM	GLYCAEMIC INDEX	SERVING SIZE (G)	EFFECT ON BLOOD GLUCOSE AS COMPARED TO ONE 4G TEASPOON OF SUGAR	
Basmati rice	69	150	10.1	✓✓✓✓✓✓✓✓✓✓
Boiled white potato	96	150	9.1	✓✓✓✓✓✓✓✓✓
Baked fries	64	150	7.5	✓✓✓✓✓✓✓
Boiled white spaghetti	39	180	6.6	✓✓✓✓✓✓
Boiled sweetcorn	60	80	4.0	✓✓✓✓
Boiled frozen peas	51	80	1.3	✓
Banana	62	120	5.7	✓✓✓✓✓
Apple	39	120	2.3	✓✓
Small slice wholemeal	74	30	3.0	✓✓✓
Broccoli	15	80	0.2	Other foods on the very low glycaemic range would be chicken, oily fish, almonds, mushrooms, cheese, meat
Eggs	0	60	0	

but starchy foods like bread, rice or potatoes are harder to quantify. Nevertheless, starchy foods like breakfast cereals or rice are surprisingly full of sugar. This is because the starch molecule is actually glucose molecules 'holding hands'. Digestion breaks starchy foods back down into lots of glucose. But how much?

The glycaemic index (GI) ranks the different carbohydrates in our foods against pure glucose. The glycaemic load (GL) is derived from this and gives us an answer in equivalent grams of glucose that specific portions of those foods can be expected to generate. This is the basis of the low-GI or low-carb diet: eating foods that don't put your blood glucose up is key to making better dietary choices to improve blood sugar control.

In our clinic, it became clear that neither patients nor most health care professionals understood the glycaemic index or its derived glycaemic load. We found this was due to the fact that most people are unfamiliar with both glucose and grams as a measure of weight. So, few people really understand what, say, 16 grams of glucose looks like. With my friend Dr Geoffrey Livesey (one of the original researchers into the glycaemic index), I re-interpreted the glycaemic load of specific portions of food into something far more familiar: a 4-gram teaspoon of table sugar. We published a paper on this in 2016[3], thus launching our 'teaspoon of sugar' infographics. There are seven of these now, translated into 18 languages and downloaded more than a million times. The full list is free to download here: www.phcuk.org/sugar/. Let's look at the one opposite to see how it could help you.

As you can see, just 150 grams of boiled rice (a small bowlful) can be expected to put your blood

93%[7] of those with pre-diabetes achieved a normal HbA1c

77%[8] of those who have been diagnosed with T2D within 1 year and choose to try low carb achieved drug-free remission

51%[8] of those who have been diagnosed with T2D for an average duration of 5.4 years achieved drug-free remission

sugar up to the same extent as 10 teaspoons of sugar. So not a good choice for people with type 2 diabetes. Even a small slice of brown bread is like 3 teaspoons of sugar. The good news is that there are many healthy, delicious foods that don't put your blood sugar up nearly so much. Knowing more about these low-carb foods could help you plan a much healthier diet. Which is exactly what this book is about!

A window of opportunity into better metabolic health

As we published our various papers through the years[1, 4–6], we noticed an important trend. The earlier our patients adopted a low-carb diet in their diabetic journey, the easier it was and the more likely they were to achieve a normal blood sugar level without drugs. This was not about how old they were: I have a patient aged 92 who achieved drug-free type 2 diabetes remission. It was about how long they had been struggling to deal with glucose, what I now term their 'metabolic age'. The message: going low carb is so often helpful, but you get extra value if you do it early.

A few words on gluten

Something else I have noticed over the last thirty years is the increasing number of people having problems with dietary gluten. Most people going low carb are also eating less gluten – 98% of the recipes in this book are gluten-free – because this is a general name for the proteins found in starchy grains like wheat, rye and barley. Gluten helps foods maintain their shape, acting as a glue that holds food like bread together. It is what gives dough its elasticity. A small number of people are properly allergic to gluten and are said to have Coeliac disease, but far more common is a milder intolerance resulting in problems like abdominal bloating and pain. In my case, wheat causes significant joint pain and stiffness (ensuring I don't cheat on my low-carb diet). Be sure to watch out to see if you might also have improvements from eating less gluten.

But don't I need carbs for energy?

The good news is that, rather like hybrid cars, our bodies are a 'duel fuel engine'. We can burn either glucose or fat for energy. It's a fact that fat is actually a more concentrated energy source than sugar, providing 9 calories per gram compared to 4. If this is true, why is an obese person still hungry? My average patient with diabetes weighs 100kg, or nearly 16 stone (220 pounds). Despite having more than a month's supply of energy on board as fat, they are hungry for every meal and snack. This is due to the action of the hormone insulin, which is produced by your pancreas gland. Because of its imperative to get blood sugar down, in the presence of a carb-heavy diet, insulin

blocks your ability to burn fat. This is exactly the reason that whenever I ate biscuits all day I was continually hungry, despite the fat stored in my 'middle-aged spread'. As I reduced the carbs in my diet, I was better able to become a fat burner; of the fat in both my belly and my food. For so many of my patients, this has resulted in less hunger as they start burning their own fat. This helps explain the prevalence of the related 'keto diet'.

A low-carb diet contains less than 130 grams of carbs a day, but if this is cut back further to, say, 50 or even 30 grams, nearly all your energy will come from fat. To burn fat your liver has to first convert it into ketones, which are then transported around the body and used as a good source of energy. At this point, one is said to be in a state of nutritional ketosis. Not to be confused with diabetic ketoacidosis, a dangerous and very different state sometimes found in people who cannot produce enough insulin. Intriguingly, published clinical trials demonstrate that increasing ketone availability to the brain via nutritional ketosis has a beneficial effect on outcomes in mild-to-moderate dementia[9].

So in summary, this book is about helping you plan a better diet. One that not only is tasty but also helps you either avoid or improve metabolic problems like type 2 diabetes and pre-diabetes. It's a diet I have enjoyed for over ten years now. In fact, I have come to see it as a lifestyle more than a diet. I really hope you will too!

BLOOD SUGAR ON A HIGH-CARB DAY

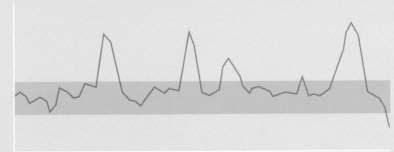

Using a continuous glucose monitor (CGM) like the Freestyle Libre means you can track changes in your blood sugar. Carby and sugary foods tend to produce a steep spike each time that food is eaten, with a return to normal levels if you have good blood sugar control.

BLOOD SUGAR ON A LOW-CARB DAY

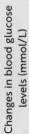
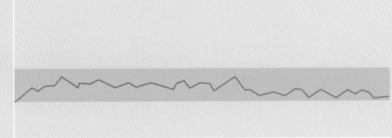

Eating low-carb goods from the recipes in this book should give you a much flatter blood glucose tracking, without the steep spikes.

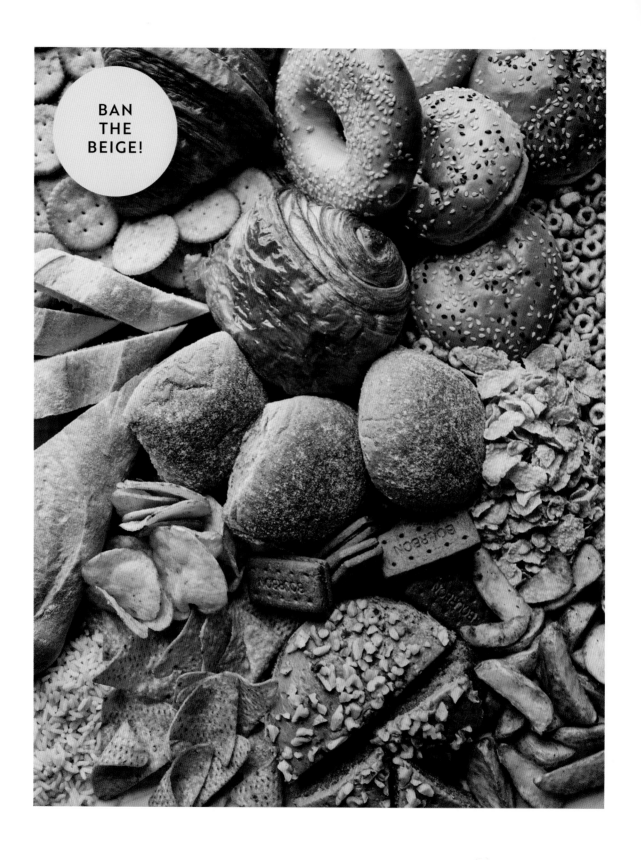

BAN
THE
BEIGE!

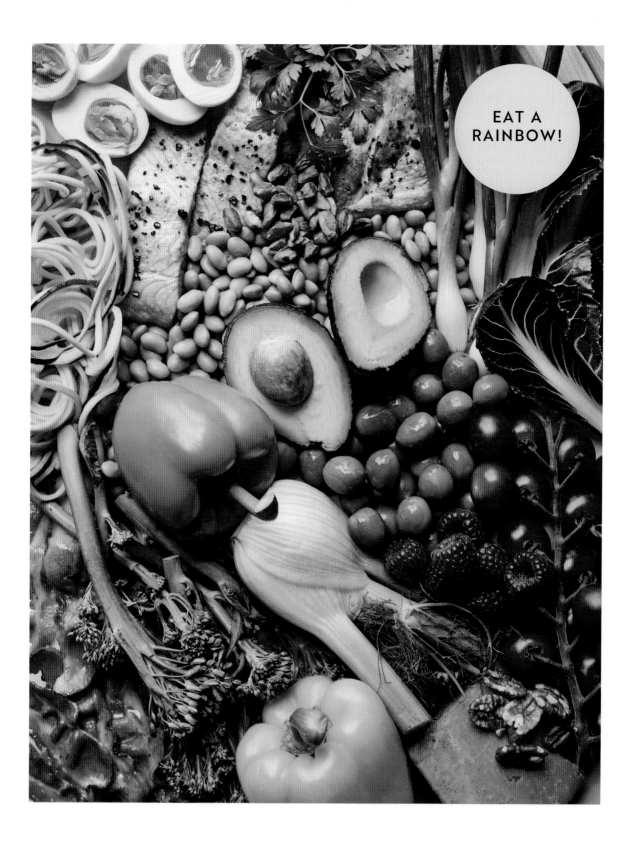

EAT A RAINBOW!

PSYCHOLOGY AND NUTRITION

Dr Jen Unwin, Clinical Health Psychologist

If eating healthily was simply a matter of knowing the right kinds of foods to eat in the right amounts, we'd all be our happy weight and feeling energized right now. Unfortunately, it is a little more complicated than that, as you have probably already realized! Just as reading the dire warnings on the sides of cigarette packets is rarely the reason people quit smoking, so overhauling our diets is more than just having the right information to hand.

Having said that, knowing the right information is the best place to start. There is so much confusion and misinformation about healthy eating at the moment. I truly believe that the knowledge you will gain from this book is the healthiest and most sustainable way to regain and retain your physical health and mental well-being long-term. I've seen innumerable people achieve health and well-being that they had given up hope of ever attaining once they started consistently applying these principles of low-carb living. Myself included. I had tried countless other nutritional plans and schemes (some a little crazy) over decades before finally finding lasting success with low-carb eating.

For so long we have been dieting and restricting, going on fad and quick-fix schemes, rather than fuelling our bodies and brains with the right nutrients they need to sustain them. Eventually our biology fights back and we find it hard to resist all the indulgent, ubiquitous 'treats',

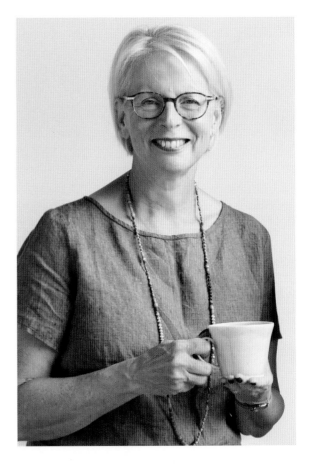

however strong-willed we are. We are condemned to a cycle of boom-and-bust eating. We have been seduced by the processed-food marketing machine into thinking that meals made in factories and labelled 'low fat' and 'healthy' are better for us than simple food cooked at home from real, fresh ingredients. We fill up on cheap cereals and giant bowls of starch that don't have the building blocks the body needs for repair. We think we need carbs for energy and to be 'fuller for longer'. We think we don't have the time or the money to live without ready meals and takeaways. I hope you will come to see, as I have, that all this is simply not true. We need to go back to first principles: which foods are proper, satisfying human foods that feed our bodies and brains? Feeding our families can, and should be, a joy and can be done simply and on a budget. More importantly, feeding ourselves and our families well is an expression of love and care that bonds us together and provides the ultimate comfort-sharing good food with those we love, so we are all full of energy for living life to the full.

Comfort food

Food can connect us at a deep level with those around us and become part of treasured family routines. Many of us can remember our favourite meals from childhood and still recreate those recipes for the next generation. We always had a roast lunch on a Sunday and looked forward to it every week. My mother would make proper chicken soup from a whole carcass when we were unwell. I had a favourite simple meal she made, called 'tuna casserole'. I would always request it on my birthday! Comfort food can be meals we associate with happy memories. In this book you will learn how some small modifications can turn comfort staples such as mashed potato or pasta into healthy low-carb alternatives that don't raise your blood sugar or lead to weight gain. We can recreate our childhood meals in healthier versions that are just as delicious and full of nutrition.

Am I a sugar addict?

Addictive food

The 'comfort' factor is not just about the associations and memories we have with certain foods. Foods high in sugars and processed grains, such as biscuits, cakes, doughnuts or pizza, quickly trigger the release of certain brain chemicals that actually change our mood. Highly palatable foods can lead to raised levels of dopamine and serotonin in the brain. These are the neurotransmitters for the feelings of reward and calmness. We really do feel *temporarily* better immediately after eating these foods! However, there is a catch. What goes up must come down. The more of these foods we eat, the more the brain cannot receive those vital chemical messages. Studies have repeatedly shown that high-sugar, refined carbohydrate and processed food diets are linked to *lower* mood and *higher* stress levels. These foods act just like other drugs such as alcohol and nicotine in the brain. Many of us have found ourselves in a trap of feeling upset or tired, treating ourselves with junk food, feeling temporary relief and then repeating the behaviour every time we feel bad, only to feel worse and worse in the long run. We have become literally addicted to processed food to feel okay.

About 20 per cent of adults and more of the younger generation now have a serious problem with ultra-processed food addiction. I have no doubt that this is what drives the current epidemics of obesity, type 2 diabetes and mental health problems. The answer is simple but not always easy in today's crazy food environment: stick to a low-carbohydrate, real-food eating plan. Cravings can soon subside if you consistently cut out these 'drug' foods. Over time, low-carb, real-food eating becomes easier, and you will notice the benefits in your mood and energy.

New habits

We are creatures of habit as well as comfort. These two are often closely intertwined. Eating in front of the TV can be a way of relaxing after work and soon becomes an ingrained habit. Buying something at the garage to snack on when you stop for fuel, having a takeaway on a Friday night, looking in the refrigerator every time you go in the kitchen; all of these can become part of our lives, not helping our long-term physical or mental health. Establishing new, desirable habits such as only eating at the table, not snacking between meals and cooking meals from fresh can take time and determination to embed. But it is worth it. Virtuous habits like brushing our teeth in the morning soon become second nature if we consistently repeat them for a while.

You will need to develop your own plan to slowly work on building good habits and dropping the harmful ones. Choose things that are relevant to you and are achievable. One idea that I have found works well is to decide on a couple of habits to work on, such as eating only at the table and taking lunch to work. Make a chart for the whole month from when you start and tick off each day you successfully carry out your new habit. Once a habit is embedded, you can add a couple of new ones to the list. They don't all need to be food related. It's important to also focus on other habits that can improve your mental well-being, so that you are less likely to reach in the biscuit barrel for comfort. Walking is a great way to boost your feel-good brain chemicals in a natural way. I take a 40 minute walk each day if I possibly can. Try it if you don't already.

	GO FOR A WALK	ONLY EAT AT THE TABLE	PACKED LUNCH
MONDAY	✓	✓	✓
TUESDAY		✓	
WEDNESDAY	✓	✓	✓
THURSDAY	✓	✓	✓
FRIDAY			✓
SATURDAY	✓	✓	
SUNDAY		✓	

Have a plan, but I want you to remember that *nobody* is perfect and there *will* be times when you struggle to keep to any plan, for example if unexpected circumstances arise or when Christmas comes around! The idea is to keep as closely as you can to the new plan each day, not to use it as a reason to berate yourself for your many failings. If one day doesn't go quite as you wish, just reset the next day. The plan is still a good one! We learn to ride a bike by wobbling and falling off. All we need to do to get better at it is keep getting back on.

Managing holidays

There are some common times when people have problems staying on plan, in my experience: weekends; birthdays; Christmas; Easter; Valentine's, Mother's or Father's Day; holidays; Halloween, etc. You see the problem! We need to learn new ways to negotiate social situations where we are inevitably faced with a festival of refined carbohydrates. These days can be every day and everywhere. I would recommend the chapter on feasts (see pages 130–153) if you are planning to host social events. Planning ahead is key and can make all the difference in staying on track. Focus on the company and the event, not the associated sugar-laden 'foods'.

What if I end up eating more carbs than I planned?

Perfection can be the enemy of long-term progress. Don't despair if you have slip-ups. Sometimes when we trip up, it can give us our best lessons. Take a moment to reflect on what you would do differently next time to get a better outcome. Get back on that bike. I have learned many useful things by messing up over the years! If you are travelling, take some emergency food. We take precooked meat and hard-boiled eggs with us on trains and planes all the time. Most supermarkets sell precooked chicken thighs, two of which make a reasonable lunch. Choose your restaurants wisely; you can usually check out menus online before you go. If you are going to a buffet party, take a plate of cold meats and a salad bowl, so you know there will be something you can eat. Most hosts and hostesses are happy if you arrive with an offering. If you are not sure when or what you will be fed, make sure you have a good meal before you set off. All of these lessons I have learned from having made bad choices because I wasn't prepared. I'm still learning lessons after ten years of living low carb. You won't have 'failed'; you'll have learned something. Dust yourself off and get right back on track.

You and your loved ones deserve the best physical and mental health so that you can be your best selves. Fuel your body and brain with what it needs and notice all the good things that come from that. And definitely don't accept that the only way to have fun is to overindulge in ultra-processed foods that will slowly rob you of the joy.

WE ARE WHAT WE EAT

Jenny Phillips, Nutrition Coach
www.inspirednutrition.co.uk

An overused phrase, maybe, but one that is hard to argue with! Save for the odd knee or hip replacement, all of our body is generated from the foods that we eat – from individual cells to organs like our liver and brain, from our bones to our skin and hair. It's remarkable when you think about it! The most powerful approach to health now is to acknowledge this fact and eat in a way that sustains and energizes us.

Low carb is a way of eating that does exactly this, and once you've grasped the principles, it can fit into most lifestyles, no matter how busy you are. I'll explain more about what we mean by low carb and 'how low you should go' on page 38 where we discuss the CarbScale.

From the point of view of managing type 2 diabetes, low carb means eating to avoid swings in your blood sugars. What does this mean? Carbohydrates are one of three macronutrients that we get from our food, the other two, I'm sure you know, are fats and protein. High carbohydrate foods include cereals, breads, pasta, rice, oats and other grains, which are also known as 'starchy carbs', and the wide range of sweet and sugary foods that are so widely available. Biscuits, cakes, sweets, chocolate, crisps and many other snack foods you may encounter contain a lot of carbohydrates. As a rough rule of thumb, consider high carb to be any food with 20g (¾oz) or more carbs per 100g (3½oz), so a quick look at the nutritional information on the packaging will alert you to this.

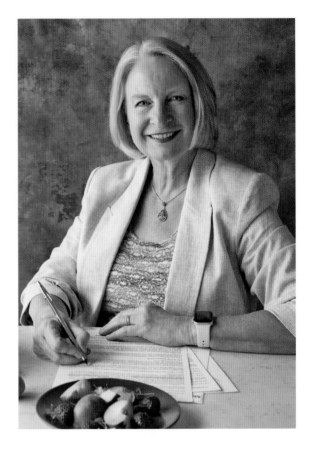

Although most people with type 2 diabetes are aware that eating sweet foods and sugar increases their blood sugars, and are advised to avoid these, they may not know that the starchy carbs in food also break down very quickly into blood glucose and thus have the same effect.

Dr Unwin has illustrated the 'carbiness' of foods by using 'teaspoon of sugar equivalents' (see page 20), which has been a massive breakthrough in

Are you metabolically healthy?

There is a cluster of five measurements that help you and your doctor to assess your metabolic health; two of these (blood pressure and waist circumference) can simply be measured from home, while the other three can be measured from a blood test via your GP, a nutritionist or a direct-to-consumer at-home test; just search online for those in your area. This information can motivate you to commit to your health to see the numbers improve. Shown here are your target ranges. Mmol/L = millimole per litre, and mm/Hg = millimetres of mercury.

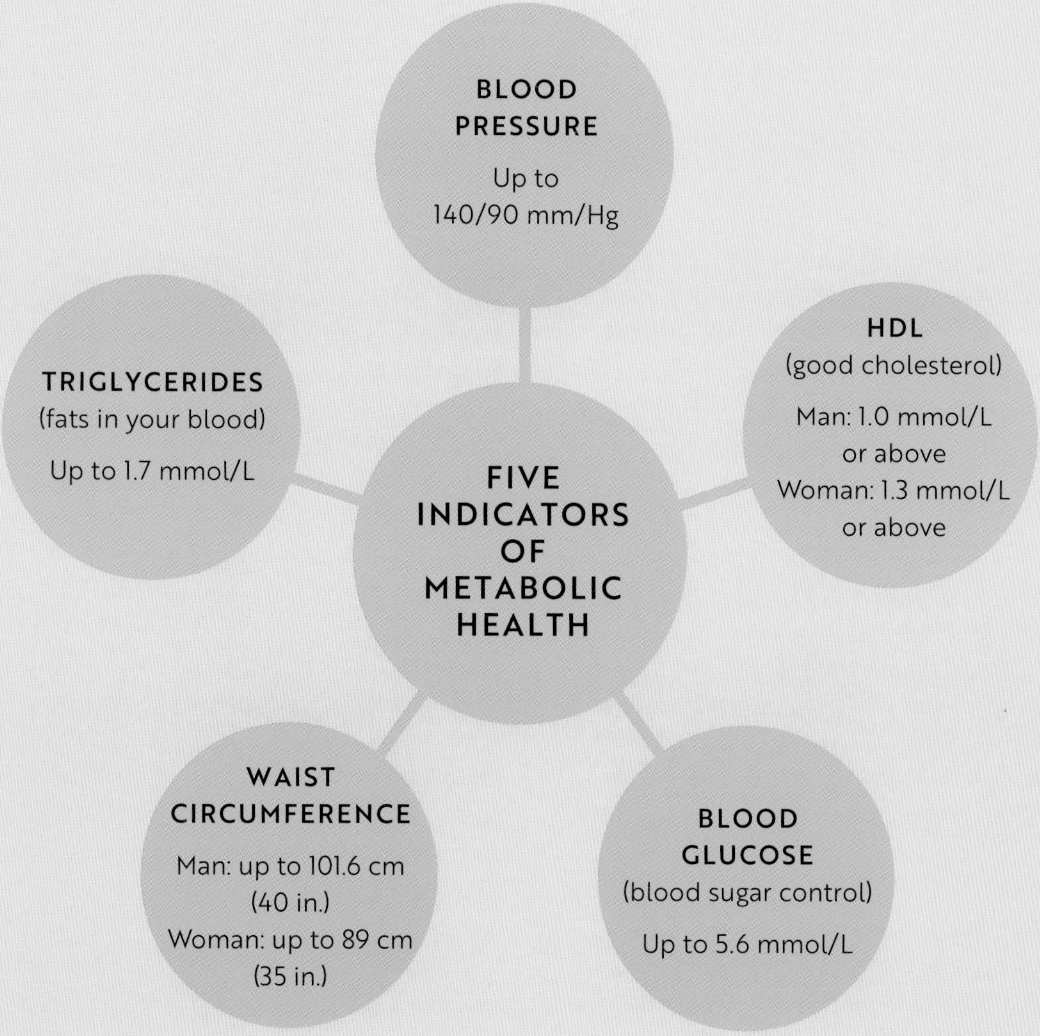

BLOOD PRESSURE

Up to
140/90 mm/Hg

HDL
(good cholesterol)

Man: 1.0 mmol/L
or above
Woman: 1.3 mmol/L
or above

TRIGLYCERIDES
(fats in your blood)

Up to 1.7 mmol/L

FIVE INDICATORS OF METABOLIC HEALTH

WAIST CIRCUMFERENCE

Man: up to 101.6 cm
(40 in.)
Woman: up to 89 cm
(35 in.)

BLOOD GLUCOSE
(blood sugar control)

Up to 5.6 mmol/L

explaining this simply. You might be quite surprised that eating a portion of rice can affect your blood sugar nearly as much as 10 teaspoons of sugar, which is why we recommend reducing or eliminating these very carby foods.

Blood sugar swings are also important to avoid if you want to lose weight and to be metabolically healthy. Having stable blood sugars from eating low-carb foods can help you feel less hungry, which means you should find it easier to control your eating. We've illustrated this on pages 34 and 36, where we compare the effect over a day of eating high-carb versus low-carb choices.

Metabolic health means that your body is functioning well and is less likely to suffer from obesity, type 2 diabetes, heart disease, stroke, kidney problems and non-alcoholic fatty liver disease. Again, low-carb eating can help all of the measurements (see previous page).

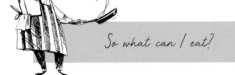

So what can I eat?

At this stage, if carbohydrates are a big part of your life, you may be feeling confused about what you can eat. The point of this book is to show you another way, with low-carb adaptations of your favourite foods and new ways to think about food.

Food for a low-carb diet

Here's what you can eat on a low-carb diet (see also the low-carb meal planner on page 42 for more detail and a simple overview of how to construct your meals):

Protein – This is the most important macronutrient for repair and muscle growth: it provides the amino acids that are the building blocks of your body. High-protein foods are meat, fish, eggs, dairy, including cheese and yoghurt, beans, lentils, soy, nuts and seeds. Our eating plans aim for a minimum of 60g (2oz) protein a day. (This is not the same as 60g/2oz of chicken, as even meat is only 20–30 per cent protein!)

Vegetables – These add colour, vitamins, minerals, fibre and variety and can really bulk out your meals so that you feel full. See page 12 for more about fibre. Dr Unwin likes to say, 'Turn your beige foods green,' meaning, 'Replace the carbs with vegetables.' For example, use cauliflower rice (see page 156) and courgetti (see page 107) in place of pasta.

Fruit – If you are trying to reverse type 2 diabetes, you may prefer to stick to low-sugar fruits like berries. If you are higher up the CarbScale (see page 38), then you may choose to add a wider range. Eating fruit with or after meals can slow the blood sugar impact. Unless you are doing a lot of exercise, you might like to limit fruit to two or three pieces a day. And always eat the whole fruit, not juice: apple or orange juice has comparable amounts of sugar to fizzy drinks!

Good fats – By reducing your calorie intake from copious carbohydrates, you have more scope to increase your fat intake without gaining, or even while losing, weight. Fats can be used to make energy to keep you active. If you eat fewer calories than you need and your body is used to burning fat as fuel, it can simply switch to burning body fat, which is the very essence of weight loss. In this way you can lower your calories without feeling hunger as your body gets all the calories it needs by 'living off the land', i.e., burning body fat as fuel.

Low-carb alternatives – This book is crammed full of different options to replace regular carbs, such as using nuts and seeds to make your own bread, crackers and even pizza base (see the baking chapter on page 170–185).

Sticking to the plan

I mention above that a benefit of the low-carb eating plan is that your hunger and cravings can quite dramatically reduce, helping you to lose weight, if you need to, without too much discomfort. But this does mean focusing on main meals and avoiding the snacks, treats and drinks that are often the real culprit in weight gain. For this reason, I ask my clients on a weight loss plan to weigh themselves twice weekly, Monday and Friday, as it is a common trend to stick more to the plan during the week and lose a few pounds, then at the weekend have a blow-out meal with pudding and wine, or other extra treats while in relaxation mode, which can cause quite a dramatic rebound of weight. If you are healthy and at your ideal weight, this may not be a problem, but for weight loss or improving your metabolic health, it just means you get stuck in maintenance and are not able to progress as you had hoped. Tracking your weight changes and isolating the weekend helps you to make better decisions.

A good start point is to have three meals a day, which is reflected in the meal plans on pages 44 and 47. Try to ensure at least 12–14 hours of fasting overnight, which means you eat every 5 to 6 hours; this is known as intermittent fasting. If this feels

right and you are meeting your goals, stay there, as it is a good way to plan your meals. If not, then flex the plan. If you're maintaining or need to gain weight, you may choose to add a healthy snack or extras like pudding. On the other hand, to boost weight loss you may need to occasionally fast for longer and eat just one or two meals a day. Remember, while you are not eating, you are 'living off the land' and burning body fat for calories.

As you flick through the pages, it will become obvious that low carb is about spending time in the kitchen and making good-quality food from fresh ingredients. A couple of points here:

– By preparing in advance and using our tips on batch cooking and storage, we hope you can accommodate enough meal prep to make low carb work for you.

– Freshly prepared food is infinitely better than ultra-processed foods (UPF) which have encroached into our shopping baskets and our kitchens.

How do you know if a product is ultra-processed? Read the back label. In a nutshell a UPF is one that includes ingredients you wouldn't find in a standard kitchen. This might include stabilizers, E numbers, additives, preservatives and more.

When you cook from scratch using ingredients, learning some meal prep tips along the way to help make things a little easier, you are looking after your health as well as providing delicious meals which friends and family can also share.

A typical day on the Western diet

BREAKFAST
Porridge with semi-skimmed milk, 50g (1¾oz)
raspberries, 200ml (7fl oz) orange juice
= 48g carbs, 13g protein, 289 kcals

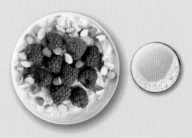

SNACK
1 banana
= 17g carbs, 1g protein, 69 kcals

LUNCH
Chicken and salad sandwich,
25g (1oz) crisps, apple
= 72g carbs, 30g protein, 547kcals

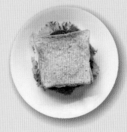

SNACK
3 chocolate biscuits
= 35g carbs, 4g protein, 279 kcals

DINNER
Lasagne, garlic bread, choc ice
= 89g carbs, 43g protein, 1109 kcals

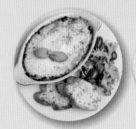

How it Affects Your Body

This is a pretty typical food diary from someone eating according to the health guidelines, which in the UK recommends eating between 2,000 (for a woman) and 2,500 (for a man) calories a day and 250–312g (9–11oz) of carbohydrates. This is the way Giancarlo used to eat when he was overweight, tired and diabetic. Each meal or snack caused a surge in his blood sugar up to levels of 15mmol/L, and his overall HbA1C at diagnosis was 79mmol/mol.

What happens to my blood sugar when I eat lots of carbohydrates?

Even if you are not diabetic, your blood sugars increase or spike with carbs. In normal circumstances, your pancreas responds by pumping out insulin, bringing down your blood sugars to safe levels. The drop in sugar can make you feel tired and hungry, and you end up on a blood sugar rollercoaster (see page 23). Insulin takes sugar into the cells to make energy or into storage, as glycogen in your liver and muscles. Any excess is converted to fat by your liver and stored in your fat cells, often around your middle. If you have belly fat, chances are it is from sugar storage!

If you have type 2 diabetes, you produce insulin but it doesn't work as well. **This is known as Insulin Resistance**. Hence blood sugar levels peak but stay high, and in addition to gaining weight, you risk other health issues, as the high sugar causes damage to the eyes, kidneys, heart and blood vessels. Over time, the pancreas may become damaged and insulin levels reduce; at this stage, your condition has progressed.

On a high-carb diet like the one opposite, you are flooding your body with sugar on a regular basis. You may even be drinking your sugar; a pint of beer has 17g (⅔oz) of carbs and a can of cola has 35g (1¼oz). Assuming each 5g (⅛oz) of carbs breaks down to approximately 1 teaspoon of sugar*, this is over 3 and 7 teaspoons per drink. Remember your blood only holds 1 teaspoon of glucose at any one time!

How can I measure my blood glucose levels?

Aside from regular blood tests or test strips, you can measure your blood sugar levels with a continuous glucose meter (CGM). You apply the device to your arm and can collect readings via a smartphone. We use the Freestyle Libre, which can be purchased online, and gives you a continuous blood sugar graph over 14 days.

What else can make my blood sugars spike?

While foods with starchy carbs or sugar are the main culprit in causing high blood sugars, there are three more circumstances in which your blood sugar could spike even without eating. The sugar comes either from glycogen stores or from breaking down protein (from muscle). Your blood sugars may rise:

- (If you have type 2 diabetes) in the morning before eating. This is known as the Dawn Phenomenon.
- When you're under stress
- With heavy exercise, such as high-intensity training

*This is a very rough-and-ready calculation. The teaspoon of sugar charts calculated by Dr Unwin are accurately derived from the glycaemic index (GI). However, the GI is not readily available for combinations of foods and recipes, or when you are in the supermarket. The 5g (⅛oz) of carbs per teaspoon correlates reasonably well with starchy carbs, most of which have a GI around or above that of table sugar (GI=65). Exceptions are pasta, which has a GI of around 42 and some fruits (e.g. an apple, which has a GI of 39) and are overstated by this calculation.

A typical day on the low-carb diet

BREAKFAST

Ginger and cinammon seed
porridge (page 54), cup of black tea

= 18g carbs, 11g protein, 440 kcals

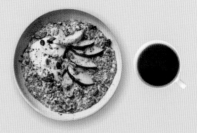

LUNCH

Ham and salad sandwich
in low-carb bread roll (page 175)
with berries

= 14g carbs, 25g protein, 446 kcals

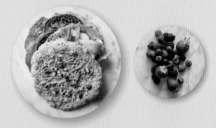

DINNER

Lamb ragu with swoodles and Parmesan
(page 106), Mango ice cream (page 193),
glass of red wine

= 23g carbs, 43g protein, 975 kcals

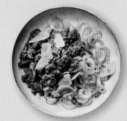

How it Affects Your Body

In contrast to a typical day eating the Western diet (see page 34), you can clearly see how making different choices can dramatically decrease your dependence on starchy carbs, all of which quickly break down to sugar. When you eat like this, wonderful things can happen. Firstly, blood sugars consistently become lower and more stable, if they were too high to begin with. This not only helps to protect you from the ravages of type 2 diabetes, but you feel amazing, too – better energy; the ability to lose weight without hunger, if you need to; and often, people report, better digestion, clearer skin and a happier mood. Using this diet, Giancarlo brought his type 2 diabetes into remission, and feels 10 years younger!

But if I don't eat carbs, what happens to my blood sugars! Will I crash??

No. Carbs, though fine for an energy source in moderation if you are fit, well and active, are not an essential food group. Yes, you need calories for energy, but these can easily be supplied by fat, which boasts 9kcals per gram versus carbs, at 4kcals per gram.

If you eat modest carbs, for example, a piece of fruit alongside a meal, you will likely see a small rise and fall of blood glucose at meal times. If you eat very low carb, or even when fasting, blood sugars typically stay flat and in the normal range. At this time you are powered by fat calories, either those you've eaten or from your fat stores, without the surges in insulin that give the boom-and-bust blood sugar curve.

If you are taking insulin-based medications, you must discuss any diet change with your doctor, as combining low carb and insulin could result in significant glucose drops. You can read more on our website TheGoodKitchenTable.com, including an excellent paper to discuss with your doctor (Campbell et al).

But what about fibre?
Will low carb make me constipated?

Low carb restricts or eliminates grains that have high fibre and are thought to improve bowel movements (although there is research to show that this can have the opposite effect in some people…). On a low-carb diet, you should be eating lots of vegetables, which also provide lots of fibre and variety to keep your gut microbiome, the good bacteria that keep you healthy, well fed.

Some foods are particularly good for prebiotics, food for the good guys, and low-carb options include: onions, leeks, garlic, asparagus, artichokes, apples, konjak root (used in low-carb noodles), and flax and chia seeds. For a really good prebiotic breakfast, try Katie's Raspberry, Chia and Oat Pots (see page 53).

You could also try adding probiotic foods to your diet, for example, live natural yoghurt, sauerkraut and kimchi, but be sure to avoid those that have been pasteurized, as this destroys the good bacteria (or you could make your own!).

Managing your carbs

This book is a low-carb, not a no-carb, meal planner, as it would be difficult to cut out all starchy carbs without excluding all fruits and vegetables. The CarbScale allows you to manage your carb intake depending on your health goals and helps you to flex how you eat.

Overall, low carb is considered up to around 130g (4½oz) carbs a day, which is half or more of what many people eat. Unless you are a very active sports person, then this should give you a good range to work to. You can flex your carb intake according to your health goals.

How low should you go? The CarbScale

1. You have type 2 diabetes and/or want to lose weight – Keep your carbs very low – 30–50g (1–1¾oz) per day – to help stabilize your blood sugars. If you don't need to lose weight, you will need to significantly increase your fat intake to ensure that you eat sufficient calories, from avocados, nuts, seeds, olive oil, dairy and the natural fats in fish and meats.

2. You want to lose weight – Again, keep quite low, 50–75g (1¾oz–2½oz) of carbs per day, to help you to lose weight, provided that you reduce your overall calories. Eating less often, firstly by stopping snacking between meals, is a good first step.

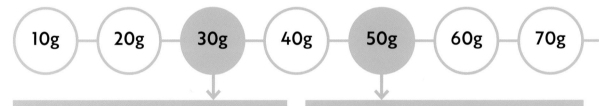

| 10g | 20g | 30g | 40g | 50g | 60g | 70g |

Keto

30–50g (1–1¾oz) carbs a day
- No grains like bread, rice and pasta
- Minimal fruit – only berries
- Minimal starchy vegetables like carrots
- Non-starchy vegetables

Strict low carb

50–75g (1¾oz–2½oz) carbs a day
- No grains like bread, rice and pasta
- Fruit two to three times a day
- Starchy (root) vegetables, excluding potato/ sweet potato
- Lots of non-starchy vegetables

As you improve your metabolic health by eating well and exercising, you may find that you can move up to higher carb levels, and then flex back as and when you need to. However, if you have been diagnosed with diabetes, you may find that avoiding the 'carb creep' altogether is the best way to keep your blood sugars stable.

If you take medication, please ensure that you discuss with your doctor before making any changes to your diet.

3. You want the benefit of good energy without the dips that carbs can cause, but are not diabetic or overweight – Flex between 75g (2½oz) and 100g (3½oz) a day, dropping lower if you need to lose a few pounds, to maintain your weight.

4. You are fit, healthy and active and have a better tolerance to carbohydrates – Have up to 130g (4½oz) a day while maintaining increased energy levels.

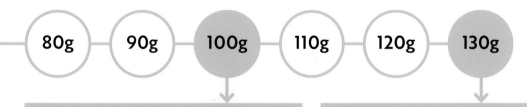

Moderate low carb

75–100g (2½–3½oz) carbs a day
- Occasional grains – rye or sourdough bread, small portions of oats, pasta or quinoa
- Fruit up to three times a day
- Starchy (root) vegetables, plus occasional potato/sweet potato (not with grains)
- Lots of non-starchy vegetables

Liberal low carb

130g (4½oz) carbs a day
- Grains most days – rye or sourdough bread, small portions of oats, rice, pasta or quinoa
- Fruit up to three times a day
- Starchy (root) vegetables, including potato/sweet potato (not with grains)
- Lots of non-starchy vegetables

Counting your carbs and calories

You may not need to. Just using the principles described in the CarbScale on page 38 may be enough to get you in the right place. However, if you find that your blood sugars stay high or your weight loss plateaus, it may be helpful to delve a little deeper. Or if you're just genuinely interested in where the carbs and calories live, counting them can be a useful learning exercise. For example, you may not know that seafood is very high in protein, while lentils have much less protein.

Fortunately, many apps are now available that help you to count the nutritional value of your food, should you want to. We particularly like Carbs & Cals (see below right), and there are many others on the market like MyFitnessPal or Nutracheck.

All the recipes in this book meet the criteria of low carb and contain full nutrition information, which can easily be used with an app. Simply make an entry for a 'new food' and enter the data provided here. For extra foods just search the app's database. If you don't have an app to refer to, you can, of course, record information in a notebook instead, and just search online for the nutrition information about your foods.

Do remember, though, to account for everything that passes your lips (including drinks containing calories). You might be surprised at how many calories slip in between meals....

The purpose of capturing more information is to make better decisions so that you can meet your own health goals.

Low carb foods
Under 10g (⅓oz) per 100g (3½oz)
Meat, fish, eggs, cheese, yoghurt, cream, butter, nuts, seeds, olive oil, non-starchy vegetables.

Medium carb foods
10–20g (¼–¾oz) per 100g (3½oz)
Lentils, beans, fruit, quinoa, starchy (root) vegetables.

High carb foods
Over 20g (¾oz) per 100g (3½oz)
Bread, oats, dried fruit, pasta, rice, potato/sweet potato.

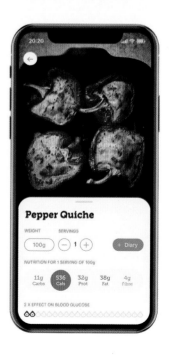

Know what you are eating

Is your food nutrient-dense or energy-dense?

Real foods such as eggs, cheese, red meat, fish or leafy greens are naturally nutrient-dense and minimally altered from their natural state. They are full of nutrients, will fill you up and nourish you. Fake food, such as sugary drinks and sweets, and starchy foods, like savoury snacks in packets and biscuits, are far from their natural state. They usually contain sugar and highly processed oils; they may provide instant energy (which you don't need if you're sitting at a desk), but they won't nourish you.

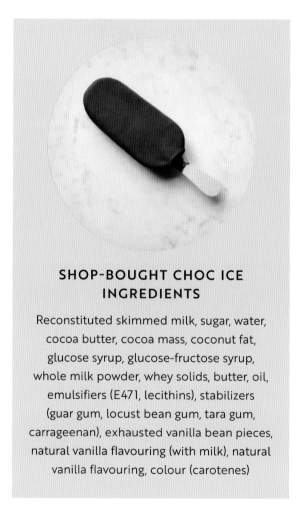

SHOP-BOUGHT CHOC ICE INGREDIENTS

Reconstituted skimmed milk, sugar, water, cocoa butter, cocoa mass, coconut fat, glucose syrup, glucose-fructose syrup, whole milk powder, whey solids, butter, oil, emulsifiers (E471, lecithins), stabilizers (guar gum, locust bean gum, tara gum, carrageenan), exhausted vanilla bean pieces, natural vanilla flavouring (with milk), natural vanilla flavouring, colour (carotenes)

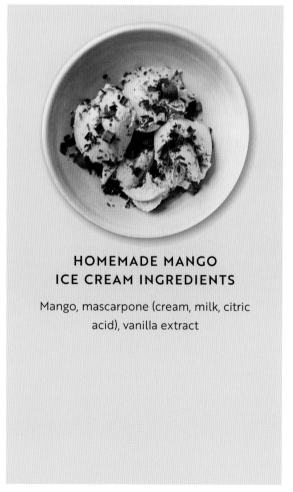

HOMEMADE MANGO ICE CREAM INGREDIENTS

Mango, mascarpone (cream, milk, citric acid), vanilla extract

Low-carb meal planner

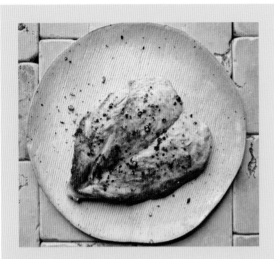

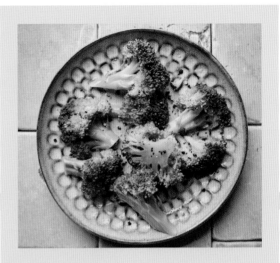

Choose your protein

Protein content given for 100g (3½oz) of each item

High protein: canned sardines, drained (22g), Cheddar cheese (26g), cod or haddock (24g), goat's cheese (22g), halloumi (24g), 2 high-meat-content sausages (21g), lamb's liver (30g), lean lamb steak (28g), lean sirloin steak (34g), pork chop (24g), salmon steak (23g), turkey or chicken breast (35g)

Medium protein: Feta cheese (16g), lentils (10.6g), 2 medium eggs (16g), peeled prawns (14g), tofu (12.6g)

Lower protein: Chickpeas (7.2g), cottage cheese (7.2g), full-fat Greek yoghurt (5.6g)

Nuts and seeds: flaxseed (6.6g), hemp seeds (11g), pumpkin seeds (8.6g), sunflower seeds (7g), whole almonds (6g)

+Vegetables

Asparagus, aubergine, artichoke, broccoli, Brussels sprouts, cabbage, cauliflower, celeriac, celery, courgette, cucumber, fennel, garlic, green beans, kale, leek, lettuce, mangetout, mushroom, okra, olives, onion, peas, pepper, pumpkin, radish, rocket, runner beans, spinach, swede, tomato, turnip, watercress

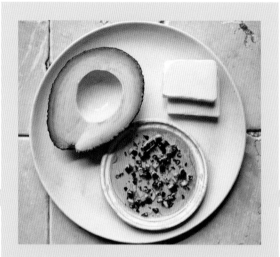

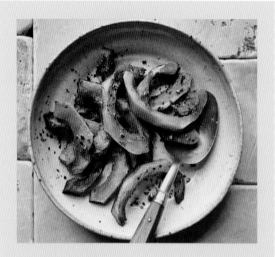

+Healthy fats

Avocado, butter, coconut oil, ghee, nuts, olive oil, seeds

Mayonnaise, gravy, vinaigrette, green goddess sauce or any of the sauces from the Sauces & Dips chapter

+More carbs

If you are higher on the CarbScale (page 38)

Starchy vegetables: Beetroot, butternut squash, carrot, parsnip, potato, sweetcorn, sweet potato

Medium-sugar fruits: Apple, apricot, nectarine, peach, pear, plum, pomegranate,

Although these are good for you, consume in moderation.

High-sugar fruits: banana, dried fruit such as raisins or dried apricot, mango, melon, watermelon.

These can cause blood sugar to spike.

Weekly meal plan for weight loss

This plan averages 1,511 kcals, 36g carbs and 81g protein a day. You can see nutritional info for each meal and additional meal plans at our website, www.thegoodkitchentable.com.

This meal plan includes a fasting period on Sunday morning. For more information about fasting see page 33.

	BREAKFAST	LUNCH	DINNER	
SATURDAY	Green shakshuka (p. 60)	Tomato and pepper soup (p. 78)	Steak (p .102), Herb butter (p. 66), Crunchy aubergine chips (p. 157), Peach and hazelnut tart (p. 194), 175ml (6fl oz) wine	Carbs: 24g Protein: 101g Cals: 1,621 kcals
SUNDAY	*Fast*	Blueberry and lemon pancakes (p. 57), yoghurt	Pulled pork (p. 146), Roasties (p. 166), Coleslaw alla Unwin (p. 161), Hot raspberry sponge pudding (p. 199), Vanilla custard (p. 200)	Carbs: 47g Protein: 83g Cals: 1,523 kcals
MONDAY	Pink yoghurt (p. 50)	Chive and smoked Cheddar omelette (p. 81), tomato	Leftover Pulled pork (p. 146), Roasties (p. 166), Coleslaw alla Unwin (p. 161)	Carbs: 34g Protein: 92g Cals: 1,509 kcals
TUESDAY	Pink yoghurt (p. 50)	Cobb salad (p. 88)	Smash bacon cheese burger (p. 99), mixed salad, vinaigrette (p. 66)	Carbs: 33g Protein: 81g Cals: 1,536 kcals
WEDNESDAY	Ginger and cinnamon seed porridge (p. 54), yoghurt, apple	Rustic roll (p. 175) with ham and salad, berries	Swoodles with Lamb ragu (p. 106)	Carbs: 49g Protein: 77g Cals: 1,530 kcals
THURSDAY	Raspberry, chia and oat pots (p. 53)	Pizza aubergines (p. 83), mixed salad, vinaigrette (p. 66)	Salmon and asparagus traybake (p. 94)	Carbs: 25g Protein: 64g Cals: 1,357 kcals
FRIDAY	Raspberry, chia and oat pots (p. 53)	Pepper quiches (p. 87), apple	Oven-baked seabass fillets with a lemon cream sauce (p. 97), courgetti (p. 107)	Carbs: 43g Protein: 67g Cals: 1,502 kcals

Weekly meal plan for weight loss, vegetarian

This plan averages 1,469 kcals, 59g carbs and 61g protein a day. You can see nutritional info for each meal and additional meal plans at our website, www.thegoodkitchentable.com.

	BREAKFAST	LUNCH	DINNER	
SATURDAY	Green shakshuka (p. 60)	Tomato and red pepper soup (p. 78), Rustic roll (p. 175)	Layered mushroom, goats' cheese, pepper and celeriac pie (p. 142), broccoli, 175ml (6fl oz) wine, Peach and hazelnut tart (p. 194)	Carbs: 56g Protein: 54g Cals: 1,546 kcals
SUNDAY	Blueberry and lemon pancakes (p. 57), yoghurt	Tomato and red pepper soup (p. 78), apple	Moussaka (p. 127), green beans and cherry tomatoes (p. 158), Za'atar flatbread (p. 178), raspberries with single cream	Carbs: 74g Protein: 49g Cals: 1,418 kcals
MONDAY	Pink yoghurt (p. 50)	Chive and smoked Cheddar omelette (p. 81), tomato	Moussaka (p. 127), green beans and cherry tomatoes (p. 158), Za'atar flatbread (p. 178), raspberries with single cream	Carbs: 54g Protein: 64g Cals: 1,507 kcals
TUESDAY	Ginger and cinnamon seed porridge (p. 54), yoghurt, apple	Cobb salad (p. 88)	Leftover Layered mushroom, goats' cheese, pepper and celeriac pie (p. 142), Chocolate, date and walnut brownie (p. 188)	Carbs: 67g Protein: 59g Cals: 1,567 kcals
WEDNESDAY	Ginger and cinnamon seed porridge (p. 54), yoghurt, apple	Rustic roll (p. 175) with 2 eggs and salad, berries	Leek paccheri with cheesy bean sauce (p. 110)	Carbs: 64g Protein: 51g Cals: 1,433 kcals
THURSDAY	Raspberry, chia and oat pots (p. 53)	Pizza aubergines (p. 83), mixed salad, vinaigrette (p. 66)	Spicy root patties and eggs (p. 84)	Carbs: 40g Protein: 65g Cals: 1,389 kcals
FRIDAY	Raspberry, chia and oat pots (p. 53)	Pepper quiches (p. 87), apple	Spicy root patties and eggs (p. 84)	Carbs: 55g Protein: 82g Cals: 1,424 kcals

Weekly meal plan for maintenance

This plan averages 1,838 kcals, 47g carbs and 88g protein a day. You can see nutritional info for each meal and additional meal plans at our website, www.thegoodkitchentable.com.

	BREAKFAST	LUNCH	DINNER	
SATURDAY	Green shakshuka (p. 60)	Tomato and red pepper soup (p. 78), Rustic roll (p. 175)	Steak (p. 102), Herb butter (p. 66), Crunchy aubergine chips (p. 157), Peach and hazelnut tart (p. 194), 175ml (6fl oz) wine	Carbs: 30g Protein: 114g Cals: 1,969 kcals
SUNDAY	Blueberry and lemon pancakes (p. 57), yoghurt	Tomato and red pepper soup (p. 78), apple	Pulled pork (p. 146), Roasties (p. 166), Coleslaw alla Unwin (p. 161), Hot raspberry sponge pudding (p. 199), Vanilla custard (p. 200)	Carbs: 66g Protein: 85g Cals: 1,705 kcals
MONDAY	Pink yoghurt (p. 50), granola	Chive and smoked Cheddar omelette (p. 81), tomato	Leftover Pulled pork (p. 146), Roasties (p. 166), Coleslaw alla Unwin (p. 161)	Carbs: 40g Protein: 98g Cals: 1,785 kcals
TUESDAY	Pink yoghurt (p. 50), granola	Cobb salad (p. 88)	Smash bacon cheese burger (p. 99), Crunchy aubergine chips (p. 157)	Carbs: 40g Protein: 94g Cals: 1,882 kcals
WEDNESDAY	Ginger and cinnamon seed porridge (p. 54), yoghurt, apple	Rustic roll (p. 175) with ham and salad, berries	Swoodles with Lamb ragu (p. 106), Mango ice cream (p. 193), 175ml (6fl oz) red wine	Carbs: 55g Protein: 79g Cals: 1,861 kcals
THURSDAY	Raspberry, chia and oat pots (p. 53)	Pizza aubergines (p. 83), mixed salad, vinaigrette (p. 66)	Salmon and asparagus traybake (p. 94), 2 Chocolate, date and walnut brownies (p. 188)	Carbs: 48g Protein: 72g Cals: 1,779 kcals
FRIDAY	Raspberry, chia and oat pots (p. 53)	Pepper quiches (p. 87), mixed salad, vinaigrette (p. 66)	Oven-baked seabass fillets with a lemon cream sauce (p. 97), courgetti (p. 107), Coffee ricotta shot (p. 201), 175ml (6fl oz) white wine	Carbs: 52g Protein: 73g Cals: 1,886 kcals

Weekly meal plan for maintenance, vegetarian

This plan averages 1,852 kcals, 65g carbs and 70g protein a day. You can see nutritional info for each meal and additional meal plans at our website, www.thegoodkitchentable.com.

	BREAKFAST	LUNCH	DINNER	
SATURDAY	Green shakshuka (p. 60)	Tomato and red pepper soup (p. 78), Rustic roll (p. 175), cheese	Layered mushroom, goats' cheese, pepper and celeriac pie (p. 142), broccoli, 175ml (6fl oz) wine, Peach and hazelnut tart (p. 194)	Carbs: 54g Protein: 69g Cals: 1,934 kcals
SUNDAY	Blueberry and lemon pancakes (p. 57), yoghurt	Tomato and red pepper soup (p. 78), Rustic roll (p. 175)	Moussaka (p.127), Za'atar flatbread, (p.178), Green beans and cherry tomatoes (p.158), Raspberry sponge pudding and custard (p.199)	Carbs: 71g Protein: 67g Cals: 1,906 kcals
MONDAY	Pink yoghurt (p. 50), granola	Chive and smoked Cheddar omelette (p. 81), tomato	Moussaka (p.127), Za'atar flatbread, (p.178), Green beans and cherry tomatoes (p.158), Raspberry sponge pudding and custard (p.199)	Carbs: 64g Protein: 76g Cals: 1,979 kcals
TUESDAY	Pink yoghurt (p. 50), granola	Cobb salad (p. 88)	Leftover Layered mushroom, goats' cheese, pepper and celeriac pie (p.142, Chocolate, date and walnut brownie (p.188)	Carbs: 72g Protein: 67g Cals: 1,807 kcals
WEDNESDAY	Ginger and cinnamon seed porridge (p. 54), yoghurt, apple	Rustic roll (p. 175) with 2 eggs, mayonnaise (p. 65) and salad, berries	Leek paccheri with cheesy bean sauce (p. 110), Mango ice cream (p. 193), 175ml (6fl oz) wine	Carbs: 70g Protein: 53g Cals: 1,767 kcals
THURSDAY	Raspberry, chia and oat pots (p. 53)	Pizza aubergines (p. 83), mixed salad, vinaigrette (p. 66)	Spicy root patties and eggs (p. 84), Tahini dressing (p. 70), Chocolate, date and walnut brownie (p. 188)	Carbs: 61g Protein: 73g Cals: 1,766 kcals
FRIDAY	Raspberry, chia and oat pots (p. 53)	Pepper quiches (p. 87), mixed salad, vinaigrette (p. 66)	Spicy root patties and eggs (p. 84), Coffee ricotta shot (p. 201), 175ml (6fl oz) white wine	Carbs: 64g Protein: 88g Cals: 1,808 kcals

LOW-CARB SWAP

PORTION OF CORNFLAKES

(30G/1OZ)

25G CARBS

VS

GREEN SHAKSHUKA (PAGE 60)

1 PORTION

6G CARBS

What should I have for breakfast? Throw out the sugary cereal and sweet pastries and bring in nutritious, great tasting food that won't give you a sleepy, hungry slump mid-morning. If you don't have time for breakfast, plan what to take to work or eat in a hurry. The Apple Crumble Bites, Pecan and Orange Granola or the Ginger and Cinnamon Seed Porridge are portable and delicious.

When you have a little more time, try the Green Shakshuka or make the Breakfast Wrap with a Spinach Sheet on page 121.

You will see cinnamon cropping up in this chapter as it can help to reduce blood sugar spikes, as well as chia seeds which are high in protein, low in carbs and great for a healthy digestion.

A word of warning, as I have been testing recipes I realize that leaving things out, such as a jar of granola or the Apple Crumble Bites, is not a good idea. They are too tempting to snack on, so put them away, out of sight!

BREAKFAST & BRUNCH

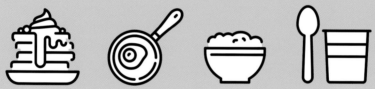

PINK YOGHURT

Serves 1

150g (5½oz) 10% fat kefir or
    Greek yoghurt
100g (3½oz) fresh, ripe or
    defrosted strawberries or
    raspberries
1 teaspoon vanilla extract
30g (1oz) roughly chopped nuts
    (optional)

PER SERVING WITH NUTS:
NET CARBS 20g | FIBRE 4g
PROTEIN 15g | FAT 28g | 370kcal

PER SERVING WITHOUT NUTS:
NET CARBS 12g | FIBRE 2g
PROTEIN 10g | FAT 11g | 206kcal

Rather than buy commercial, flavoured yoghurts that are packed with sugar, make your own by mashing berries into thick Greek yoghurt. This is a great breakfast for adults and kids, plus it is low in carbs and quick to prepare. To make it higher in protein, and therefore more substantial, add the chopped nuts, a handful of Pecan and Orange Granola from page 52 or a couple of Apple Crumble Bites (see page 58).

In a bowl, use a fork to mash the berries into the yoghurt. To give a little sweetness, add the vanilla extract and stir in. Top with the nuts, if using, and serve straight away or chill in the refrigerator for up to 2 days until you are ready to eat.

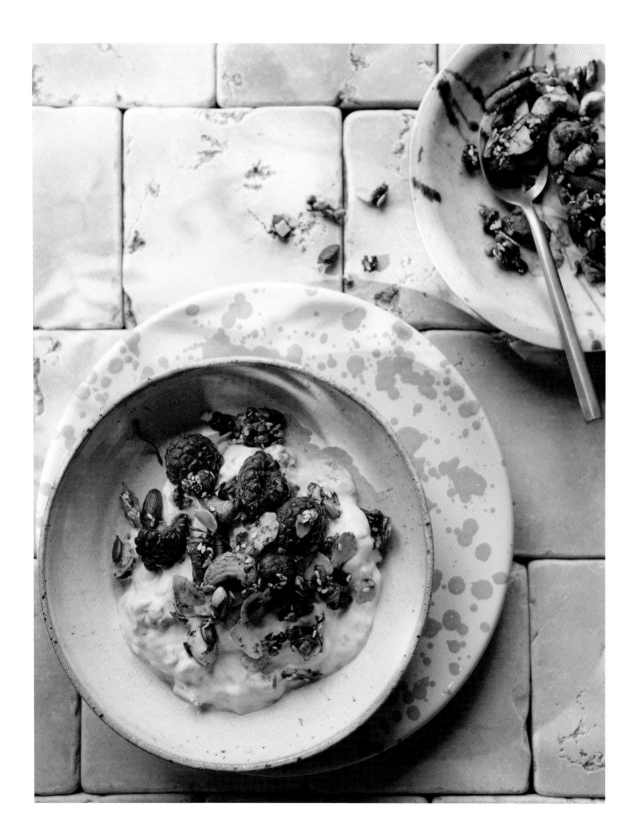

PECAN AND ORANGE GRANOLA

**Serves 6
(makes 260g/9¼oz)**

15g (½oz) unsalted butter or
    coconut oil
25g (1oz) honey or 1 heaped
    tablespoon erythritol
25g (1oz) flaked almonds
1 egg white, lightly beaten
125g (4½oz) pecans or other
    mixed nuts
75g (2½oz) mixed seeds (such as
    pumpkin, sunflower, sesame)
2 teaspoons vanilla extract
2 teaspoons ground cinnamon
finely grated zest of 1 small orange
pinch of salt

**PER SERVING (APPROX. 40G/1½OZ) WITH
ERYTHRITOL:** NET CARBS 3g | FIBRE 3g
PROTEIN 6g | FAT 26g | 263kcal

**PER SERVING (APPROX. 40G/1½OZ)
WITH HONEY:** NET CARBS 6g | FIBRE 3g
PROTEIN 6g | FAT 26g | 276kcal

Although high in calories, nuts are great for filling us up and providing insoluble fibre for our gut health, vitamins and healthy fats. Don't leave a bowl of this around, or you will find yourself snacking on it; put the granola in a jar and measure out portions as you need. Any open packets of nuts or seeds should be stored in the fridge or freezer to stop them becoming rancid. Do check them first before using as it is such a pity to make this with old ingredients; I've done it!

This tasty granola is so much healthier than the sugar-laden ones you can buy in the shops. I have used minimal honey for a hint of sweetness, but if you prefer, use erythritol instead. Over time you could completely reduce or remove the sweetness. If you don't have time for breakfast, take a serving of the dry granola to work and have it with a coffee. Otherwise, top Greek yoghurt with the granola and add a few berries. To weigh out the honey, hold a spoon in hot water briefly before spooning it out, so it will slip easily off.

Heat the oven to 200°C/180°C fan (400°F), Gas Mark 6. Line a baking tray with a silicone baking mat or silicone paper.

Melt the butter or coconut oil and honey or erythritol together in a small bowl in the microwave or in a small saucepan. Add the remaining ingredients to a larger bowl, pour in the melted butter and honey, and stir thoroughly.

Spread out the mixture on the lined baking tray and bake for 7 minutes or until the egg white has set and the nuts are lightly browned. Keep an eye on it, as nuts easily burn. Use a slice or spatula to turn the granola over in large chunks and place back into the oven for 2 minutes or until it is dry, firm to the touch and lightly browned.

Remove the granola from the oven and allow it to cool on the tray. It can be stored in a jar at room temperature for up to 3 days or in the refrigerator for a week.

RASPBERRY, CHIA AND OAT POTS

Serves 1

1 tablespoon whole white or black chia seeds

5 tablespoons water, more if you add oats

100g (3½oz) 10% fat kefir or Greek yoghurt

½ teaspoon vanilla extract

15g (½oz) roughly chopped nuts (such as almonds, walnuts or pecans)

100g (3½oz) raspberries, strawberries, blackberries or blueberries

20g (¾oz) whole oats (optional)

PER SERVING: NET CARBS 12g | FIBRE 11g PROTEIN 11g | FAT 23g | 330kcal

OPTIONAL:

20G (¾OZ) OATS: NET CARBS 13g FIBRE 1g | PROTEIN 2g | FAT 1g | 74kcal

Tiny black or white chia seeds are great for keeping you regular, adding protein and as a thickener. Left to soak in liquid, they swell and form a gel, which is great for adding body to a dish. You can leave out the nuts and yoghurt if you want to keep it simple, or add the oats for energy if you're exercising.

Stir the chia seeds into the water in a serving bowl. Leave to stand for 20 minutes, or overnight if you prefer.

Stir in the remaining ingredients, adding a little more water if using oats, and enjoy.

ANYWHERE CHIA PORRIDGE

Serves 1

For the dry mixture

1 tablespoon whole chia seeds

2 tablespoons mixed seeds (such as flax, sunflower, pumpkin)

¼ teaspoon ground cinnamon

pinch of vanilla powder

25g (1oz) pecans, almonds or walnuts, roughly chopped

20g (¾oz) oats (optional)

To serve

1 ginger tea bag, optional

½ apple

50g (1¾oz) 10% fat kefir or Greek yoghurt (optional)

PER SERVING: NET CARBS 4g | FIBRE 7g
PROTEIN 8g | FAT 30g | 326kcal

OPTIONAL:

50G (1¾OZ) GREEK YOGHURT:
NET CARBS 2.5g | FIBRE 0g
PROTEIN 2g | FAT 5g | 62kcal

½ APPLE: NET CARBS 12g | FIBRE 3g
PROTEIN 0.5g | FAT 0g | 52kcal

20G (¾OZ) OATS: NET CARBS 13g
FIBRE 1g | PROTEIN 2g | FAT 1g | 74kcal

This is a delicious hot or cold breakfast and replaces a bowl of traditional starchy porridge that would be likely to spike your blood glucose. You can prepare a larger quantity of the dry mixture in advance and store it in a jar or a bag. I take some, along with an apple, for overnight stays in hotels where I'm not sure if I'll get a healthy breakfast. I even prepare enough for a seven-day holiday abroad. I can make it up in my room and eat it from a mug! I sometimes do this the night before and leave it in the mini-refrigerator to cool overnight, which allows the seeds to swell further. Or I can take it down to breakfast and add water, yoghurt and an apple or berries. Travelling often upsets digestion and chia seeds can help your body find its natural rhythm. Make up the porridge with hot water and a herbal tea bag for extra flavour. Leave out the oats if you are keto.

Pour the dry mixture into a mug or bowl, add the tea bag, if using, and top up with enough just-boiled water to cover the mixture by a thumb's width. Leave to steep for 5 minutes to allow the seeds to swell. Discard the tea bag. Eat while warm as porridge or leave to cool. Add more hot or cold water as necessary until you have the consistency of porridge.

Cut the apple into slices; there is no need to peel it but do discard the core. (Keep the other half in the refrigerator for another day.) Add to the mug or bowl with the yoghurt, if using. Eat straight away.

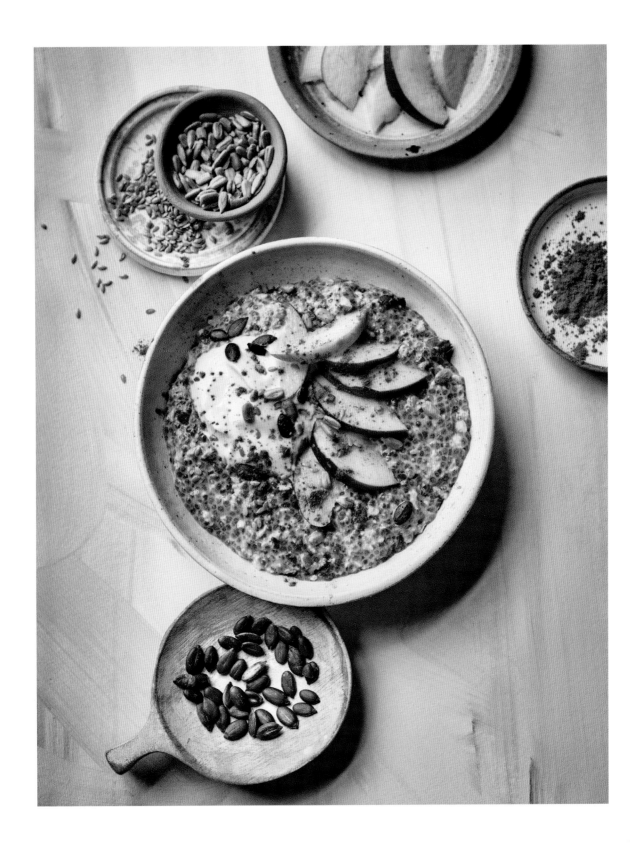

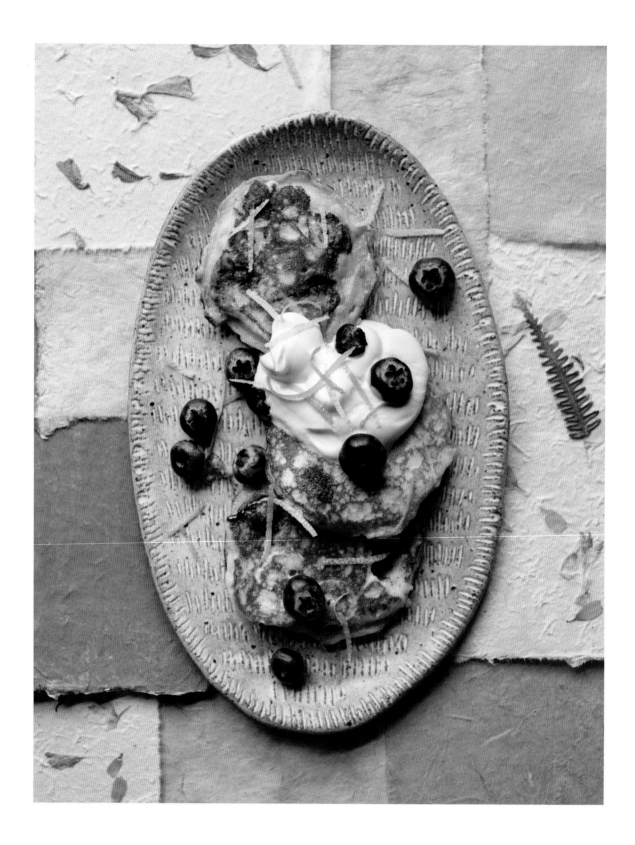

BLUEBERRY AND LEMON PANCAKES

Serves 2
(makes 6 small pancakes)

2 large eggs
1 teaspoon vanilla extract
½ teaspoon baking powder
3 tablespoons coconut flour
1 teaspoon finely grated lemon
    zest, plus extra, pared, to serve
1 tablespoon erythritol or 2
    teaspoons honey
4 tablespoons cold water
50g (1¾oz) blueberries
1 tablespoon coconut oil, ghee or
    butter, for frying
Greek yoghurt, to serve (optional)

PER SERVING USING ERYTHRITOL,
WITHOUT YOGHURT: NET CARBS 7g
FIBRE 4g | PROTEIN 9g | FAT 13g |
198kcal

PER SERVING USING HONEY, WITHOUT
YOGHURT: NET CARBS 13g | FIBRE 4g
PROTEIN 9g | FAT 13g | 218kcal

These pancakes go down a storm in our house and they have the advantage of being nut-free, gluten-free and lactose-free. They are also great with berries, yoghurt or whipped cream. You can also decide if you want to use an artificial sweetener like erythritol to lower the carbs, or keep it natural with honey. Once cooled they can be packed into containers and are good for travelling, or can be frozen. If we are at home we love them with berries and Greek yoghurt.

Whisk the eggs, vanilla, baking powder, coconut flour, lemon zest and sweetener or honey together with the water in a mixing bowl until thoroughly combined. The mixture should be thick but able to drop from a spoon: add a splash more water if necessary. Stir in the blueberries.

Heat a large, non-stick frying pan over a low–medium heat and add the coconut oil, ghee or butter. When melted and just starting to bubble, swirl the fat around the pan to coat it. Working in batches if necessary, drop 3 tablespoons of the batter into the pan to make each pancake, ensuring they don't touch as they spread out. Be patient before trying to flip them! Cook for 3–4 minutes on the first side until the edges are set and firm, then use a fish slice or spatula to gently turn the pancakes. Cook for 1–2 minutes on the second side.

Remove the pancakes from the pan and serve straight away or keep warm while you make the others. Serve as they are or with extra pared lemon on top, berries and yoghurt.

APPLE CRUMBLE BITES

Makes approx. 30 bites

75g (2½oz) pitted dates, roughly chopped, or 100g (3½oz) erythritol
4 tablespoons hot water
50g (1¾oz) chia or flaxseeds, milled
250ml (9fl oz) cold water
1 small apple
100g (3½oz) pecans or other nuts, roughly chopped
50g (1¾oz) oats
2 teaspoons vanilla extract
1 teaspoon baking powder
1 teaspoon ground cinnamon
finely grated zest of 1 small lemon or ½ orange

PER BITE WITH DATES: NET CARBS 3.5g
FIBRE 1g | PROTEIN 1g | FAT 3g | 48kcal

PER BITE WITH ERYTHRITOL:
NET CARBS 2g | FIBRE 1g | PROTEIN 1g |
FAT 3g | 40kcal

I have been asked many times to create low-carb cereal bars, but without the sugar or plenty of dates, it is hard. These bites, however, have all the flavour and chewiness of a cereal bar but contain minimal carbs. They are perfectly portable, last a long time and gradually dry further the longer they are left out, making them great for journeys or taking to work. The recipe is also gluten-free and vegan. It is cheaper to buy whole black or white chia seeds and mill them yourself until finely ground in a spice grinder or small food processor.

Line a large baking tray with baking paper.

Soak the dates, if using | in the hot water in a mixing bowl for a few minutes and then use a fork to mash them and the water to a pulp. Add the chia or flaxseeds and the cold water. Stir through; they will gradually absorb the water. If using erythritol add this to the seeds and cold water.

Cut the apple into quarters and remove just the centre woody core and stem. Cut each quarter into 4 lengthways. Then halve lengthways and cut crossways to form 5mm (¼-inch) cubes. Add to the bowl with the remaining ingredients, then thoroughly stir through.

Heat the oven to 190°C/170°C fan (375°F), Gas Mark 5.

Use a dessertspoon to drop mounds of the mixture on the lined baking tray, flattening and neatening them with the spoon as you go. They don't expand on cooking but set them apart by at least a finger width. Bake the bites for 25 minutes or until golden brown and set.

Turn the oven down to 170°C/150°C fan (325°F), Gas Mark 3. Remove the bites from the oven and use a slice to flip them over. Bake again for 8–10 minutes or until dry to the touch. Watch them carefully to make sure the nuts don't catch.

Remove from the oven and allow to cool upside down on the tray. Keep in a bowl (out of the way, so you are not tempted to snack on them) for up to 4 days or in an airtight container in the refrigerator for 10 days. They can also be frozen in a container for up to 3 months.

CHEESY SPINACH SCRAMBLE

Serves 1

2 eggs

50g (1¾oz) cooked or defrosted and well-squeezed spinach, roughly chopped

15g (½oz) Cheddar cheese, coarsely grated, or feta cheese, crumbled

pinch of salt

plenty of freshly ground black pepper

15g (½oz) butter, ghee, coconut oil or extra-virgin olive oil

Optional additions

handful of soft, roughly chopped herbs (such as coriander, basil or parsley)

pinch of chilli flakes

25g (1oz) cooked ham or bacon, roughly chopped

PER SERVING: NET CARBS 2g | FIBRE 2g PROTEIN 17g | FAT 27g | 321kcal

PER SERVING WITH HAM: NET CARBS 2g FIBRE 2g | PROTEIN 22g FAT 29g | 365kcal

I like to eat this version of scrambled eggs from a bowl with a spoon for a speedy breakfast or lunch. Adding spinach bulks up the eggs so you won't miss toast with them, just make sure you squeeze it well to get rid of any liquid. The spinach adds vitamins, iron and valuable fibre, which is great for your gut health. To add to the protein, and therefore satiety, add a slice of ham or bacon.

Beat the eggs together in a mixing bowl with a fork until they are uniform yellow. Stir in the spinach, cheese, seasoning and any additions.

Melt the butter, ghee or oil in a large non-stick frying pan over a low heat until it starts to foam. Pour in the egg mixture and stir continuously as it begins to set. Mix the runny eggs and solid areas together until it is cooked to your liking. Remove from the heat and serve straight away in a bowl on its own or on a plate with ham.

GREEN SHAKSHUKA

Serves 2

2 tablespoons extra-virgin olive oil
3 spring onions, finely chopped
¼ teaspoon ground cumin
pinch of Aleppo chilli flakes or
    finely chopped fresh chilli, plus
    extra to serve
200g (7oz) mixed green leaves
    (see recipe introduction),
    roughly chopped, or coarsely
    grated courgette
5 tablespoons water
4 eggs
100g (3½oz) feta cheese
salt and pepper

To serve
handful of coriander, leaves
    roughly torn, stems chopped
½ avocado, sliced

PER SERVING: NET CARBS 6g | FIBRE 8g
PROTEIN 23g | FAT 43g | 525kcal

This wonderful, wholesome breakfast is as nutritious as it is pretty. I love to use up whatever greens I have in the refrigerator, such as spinach, rocket, watercress or cabbage, for this. If I'm out of leaves, I defrost around 8 cubes of frozen spinach, which, once squeezed, makes around 200g (7oz) of spinach. Put the empty half of the avocado shell over the leftover one, or simply wipe it with a cut lemon, to keep it bright. I like to use Aleppo chilli flakes for their gentle flavour and bright colour.

Heat the oil in a medium frying pan (with a lid) over a medium heat, add the spring onions and fry for 5–7 minutes until soft. Add salt and pepper, cumin and chilli. Add the greens or courgette and the water to the pan. Stir through the onions and put the lid on. Cook over a gentle heat for around 5 minutes or until the greens are soft.

Remove the lid and add another 3 tablespoons of water if the first few spoons have evaporated and the mixture looks dry. Crack the eggs into the pan, and crumble over the feta. Put the lid back on and cook for 5–8 minutes or until the eggs are done to your liking.

Scatter over the coriander and add the avocado slices with a dusting of chilli. Serve straight away.

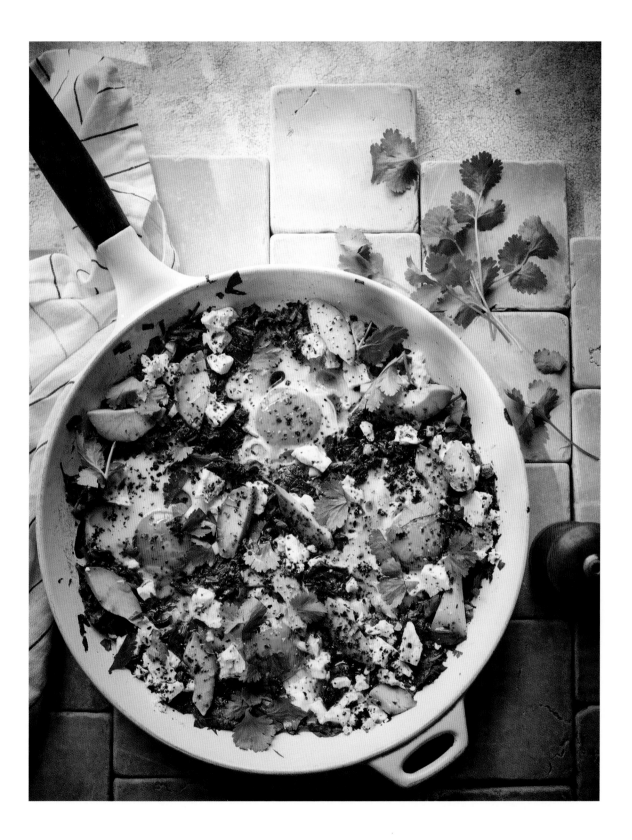

LOW-CARB SWAP

CHICKPEA HUMMUS

8G CARBS

VS

CAULIFLOWER HUMMUS (PAGE 70)

3G CARBS

After choosing the protein element of your meal, add a sauce for flavour and a dose of healthy fat. Whether the base is creamy avocado, extra-virgin olive oil or kefir yoghurt, sauces help you feel full for longer meaning you are less likely to snack.

I love to see a jar or two of homemade sauce in the fridge as then I know that a delicious meal is only minutes away. The Italian sauces in this chapter will keep for a week in the fridge and the herb butters can even be frozen.

Fresh sauces and dips sing with flavour from citrus, chilli, garlic or herbs in the way that commercial sauces don't. A spoonful of Chermoula or Romesco will bring zing to your fish or meat, the Green Chilli and Kefir dressing is sensational over salad or grilled chicken, and the Ancient Roman Cheese and Herb dip recipe is over 2,000 years old and still delights. Instead of buying ultra-processed sauces, try these easy recipes and wow your family and friends with your new prowess. By making your own you can also avoid poor-quality oils and added sugar.

SAUCES
& DIPS

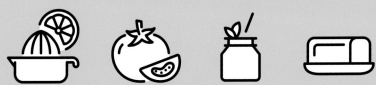

INSTANT CHEESE SAUCE

This is ridiculously quick to put together, and is delicious on everything, from steamed broccoli or cauliflower to pasta alternatives or roasted vegetables.

Serves 4

50g (1¾oz) Parmesan or Grana Padano cheese, finely grated
100ml (3½fl oz) double cream

PER SERVING:
NET CARBS 2.1g | FIBRE 0g | PROTEIN 3.9g | FAT 16g | 167kcal

Simply put the Parmesan and cream in a small pan over a low heat to melt. It will begin to bubble and thicken; stir frequently and after around 5–10 minutes, remove it when it looks like a cheese sauce and not like cream.

Even quicker is to stir the cheese into the cream in a mug and put it in the microwave for 40 seconds–1 minute until melted and thickened. Job done and ready to serve.

CLASSIC TOMATO SAUCE

If you want a classic Italian sauce and have some time, make this; it's my go-to recipe. The sauce can be blended to make it smooth, if you prefer.

Serves 6

5 tablespoons extra-virgin olive oil
1 red onion, finely chopped
1 garlic clove, lightly crushed (optional)
1 teaspoon salt
plenty of freshly ground black pepper
2 × 400g (14oz) cans Italian plum tomatoes

PER 175G (6OZ) SERVING:
NET CARBS 7g | FIBRE 4g | PROTEIN 2g | FAT 12g | 139kcal

Heat the oil in a large saucepan over a medium heat. Fry the onion and garlic, if using, for 10 minutes or until softened and translucent. Add the salt and pepper.

Add the tomatoes, then fill the cans one-quarter full with water and swill it around to collect any juices left on the sides of the cans. Add this to the pan. Bash the tomatoes with a potato masher or wooden spoon to break them up. Reduce the heat and simmer, uncovered, for around 40 minutes to concentrate the flavours; the sauce should be thick and not watery.

The sauce is ready to use straight away as it is or it can be blended. Chill and keep any leftovers in the refrigerator for up to 5 days.

> **Quick Tomato Sauce**
> For a speedier version of the above, omit the onions and fry the garlic for just 3 minutes. Continue as above but cook for just 25 minutes.
>
> Net carbs: 4g, fibre 3g, protein 1g, fat 12g, 121kcal

PESTO

Pesto is so easy to make and the results are so much better than any sauce coming out of a jar. Once you try it, you'll never look back.

Serves 8

125g (4½oz) pine nuts
50g (1¾oz) basil leaves and stalks
25g (1oz) Parmesan cheese, grated
1 small garlic clove, peeled
125ml (4fl oz) extra-virgin olive oil
salt and pepper

PER SERVING:
NET CARBS 1G | FIBRE 0.6G | PROTEIN 3.9G | FAT 26G, 257KCAL

Heat the oven to 220°C/200°C fan (425°F), Gas Mark 7.

Put the pine nuts on a baking tray and roast for a few minutes until golden brown. Remove from the oven and tip on a plate to cool.

To make the pesto, blizz the in a small foodprocessor or a pestle and mortar. Whizz or pound the ingredients together until you have either a smooth, velvety sauce or leave it textural with a crunch left to the pinenuts. Season to taste and set aside.

Serve over roast chicken or vegetables or over any of the pasta alternatives. Store the pesto in a jar in the fridge for up to 3 days.

MAYONNAISE

Take your pick of the oils in the list below, but don't be tempted to use extra-virgin olive oil in this mayo; it is too strong and bitter. Like most homemade mayonnaises, this is made with raw egg, so it isn't for pregnant women or anyone in poor health. This is the basic recipe, but you can flavour it with a little grated fresh or mashed roasted garlic, lemon zest, chopped chives, chipotle or curry powder.

Serves 4

1 medium egg
1 heaped teaspoon Dijon mustard, or more to taste
1 teaspoon lemon juice, or more to taste
½ teaspoon salt, or more to taste
good few twists of black pepper
150ml (5fl oz) avocado, cold-pressed rapeseed oil,
    macadamia or light olive oil

PER SERVING MADE WITH AVOCADO OIL:
NET CARBS 0g | FIBRE 0.5g | PROTEIN 1.9g | FAT 36g | 333kcal

Put all the ingredients into the narrow, tall mixing cup of a stick blender. If you don't have one, use a narrow, tall jam jar instead. There should be only up to 1cm (½ inch) of room around the blender stick.

Put the stick blender to the bottom and whizz for 30 seconds or until you see a thick mayonnaise forming. At that point, slowly lift the blender upward as you whizz again. Don't worry if there is a little oil left on top, you can stir this in.

Now taste the oil; at this point you can stir in more lemon juice, mustard, seasoning or other flavourings, to your taste.

It will keep for up to 3 days in the refrigerator.

VINAIGRETTE

My earliest memory of cooking is shaking the vinaigrette in a jar for my mum as she prepared salad for us all. She would get me to taste it and decide if it needed more of any of the ingredients. In that simple task she gave me surety in my taste. Thanks Mum.

Serves 8

2 tablespoons red wine vinegar or cider vinegar
8 tablespoons extra-virgin olive oil, or more to taste
2 teaspoons lemon juice, or more to taste
1 heaped teaspoon Dijon mustard
½ teaspoon honey (optional)
½ teaspoon salt, or more to taste
plenty of freshly ground black pepper
1 small garlic clove, grated (optional)

PER SERVING:
NET CARBS 1g | FIBRE 0g | PROTEIN 0g | FAT 13g | 122kcal

Put all the ingredients into a jar with a tight-fitting lid. Shake the jar until you have a creamy dressing. Taste it and add more salt, lemon or oil to your taste.

Always dress a salad just before serving and keep any remaining dressing in the refrigerator for up to a week.

Variations
Balsamic: Use a good-quality balsamic instead of the red wine or cider vinegar.

Herb: Add 2 tablespoons chopped fresh leafy herbs (such as basil, coriander, chives or parsley).

Nut: Swap half the olive oil for walnut or hazelnut oil.

Creamy: Reduce the oil by half and make up the amount with crème fraîche or double cream.

HERB BUTTER

This is great on seabass or steak (see pages 97 and 101). Now that butter is back on our menu, we love to mix it with flavourings and watch shards of it melt on hot steak or fish, spread it on warm low-carb bread or stir it into mash or scrambled eggs. Basil is my favourite flavour, while Giancarlo loves garlic, rosemary and black pepper. Chives, parsley, fresh oregano or tarragon are gorgeous, too.

Serves 4 (makes approx. 70g/2½ oz)

60g (2¼oz) salted butter, at room temperature
6g (¼oz) finely chopped fresh herbs
1 small garlic clove, grated (optional)
freshly ground black pepper

PER SERVING:
NET CARBS 0g | FIBRE 0g | PROTEIN 0g | FAT 5g | 50kcal

To make the herb butter, mix the ingredients together in a bowl, adding plenty of black pepper.

Enjoy the butter as it is or, using a dinner knife, divide the butter into four and place each quarter on a piece of baking paper. Use the knife to shape the butter into 4 shallow circles around 1cm (½ inch) deep. Cover with more paper and put in the refrigerator (or the freezer if you are in a hurry) to firm up before using. Keep in the fridge for up to 3 days or in the freezer for up to 3 months.

HOT CHILLI SAUCE

This addictively delicious sauce is so quick to whizz together and goes perfectly with roast chicken, barbecued meat, fish or vegetables, or simply drizzled over soft-boiled eggs.

Serves 8 (makes 60g/2¼oz)

1–2 red chillies
½ teaspoon chilli flakes (optional)
2 garlic cloves, peeled
6 tablespoons extra-virgin olive oil
½–1 teaspoon cider vinegar or red wine vinegar
¼ teaspoon salt
plenty of freshly ground pepper

PER SERVING:
NET CARBS 0g | FIBRE 0g | PROTEIN 0g | FAT 10g | 91kcal

Taste one of the red chillies, from the middle of the chilli where the pith joins the seeds, to see how hot they are and decide whether 1 or 2 will do the job. If neither is spicy enough, add a pinch of chilli flakes. Put all the sauce ingredients in a small food processor and whizz to combine, or finely chop by hand and mix together in a bowl. Transfer to a jug and use straight away or keep in the fridge for up to 3 days.

ROMESCO

This is a super-quick version of this wonderful Catalan sauce. The slower version involves roasting tomatoes, onions and peppers in a hot oven until they char. They are then peeled and blended with breadcrumbs. Our version omits the bread and speeds up the process by using a roasted pepper from a jar and tomato purée. Use this with white fish, chicken or on fried eggs.

Serves 6 (makes 125g/4½oz)

25g (1oz) blanched almonds
1 large roasted red pepper, from a jar
1 garlic clove, smashed
3 tablespoons extra-virgin olive oil
1 tablespoon tomato purée
1 teaspoon sherry vinegar or red wine vinegar, or more to taste
½ teaspoon smoked paprika
salt and pepper

PER SERVING:
NET CARBS 1g | FIBRE 1g | PROTEIN 1g | FAT 9g | 85kcal

Heat the oven to 220°C/200°C fan (425°F), Gas Mark 7.

Put the almonds on a baking tray and toast for around 8 minutes until lightly browned. Alternatively, toast the almonds in a dry frying pan over a medium heat for 5–10 minutes. Tip the almonds on to a plate and leave to cool.

Put the remaining ingredients into a small food processor (or use a stick blender) and blitz until very finely chopped. Taste and adjust the acidity and seasoning to your liking. Transfer to a jar; your romesco will keep in the refrigerator for up to 1 week.

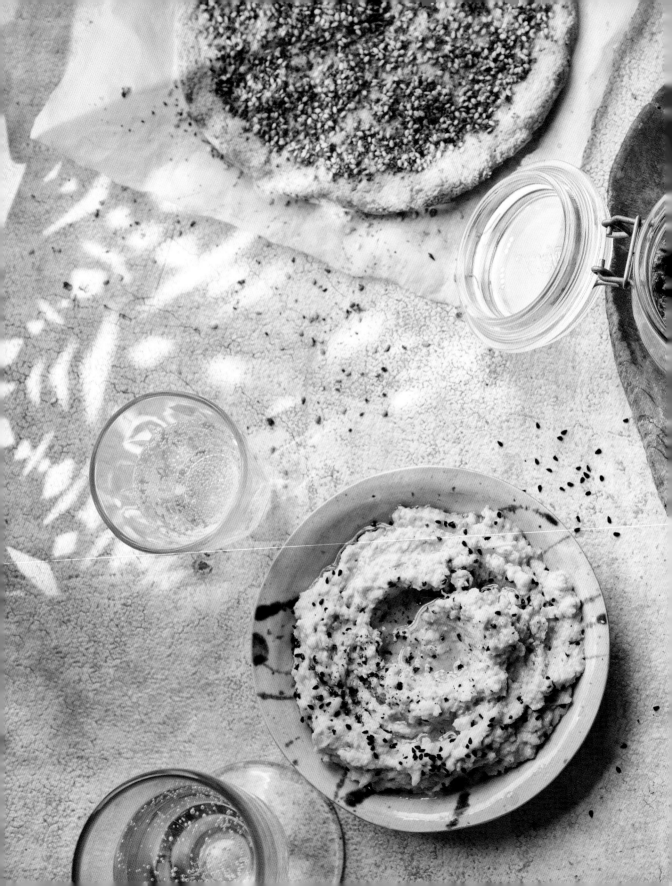

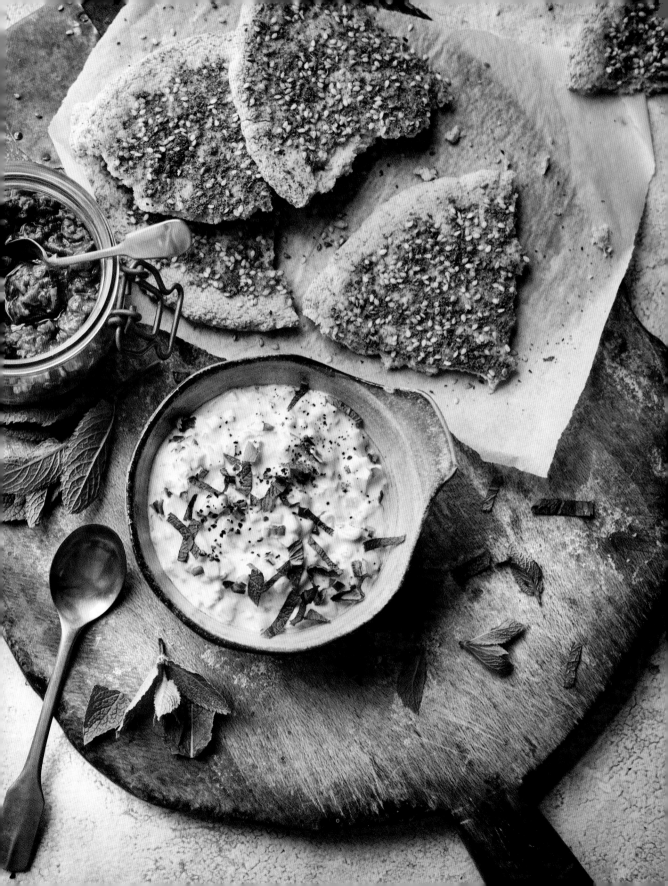

HUMMUS

I've eaten a lot of hummus developing this recipe! Cauliflower hummus is popular with those following a keto diet, and rightly so – making this recipe with chickpeas, will increase the net carbs by 5g, as compared to our friend the cauli. A powerful food processor will give the hummus a smoother finish, but any gadget that whizzes things to a purée, even a stick blender, will do. My Kuwaiti friend Amal makes a shallow base of hummus swirled on a plate, which she tops with chicken as cooked in the Cobb Salad (page 88) and fried onions; you can also try it with the Za'atar Chicken (page 105). See photo on page 68.

Serves 6

300g (10½oz) cauliflower, cut into small florets, or 260g (9¼oz) drained canned chickpeas
5 tablespoons extra-virgin olive oil, plus extra to serve
1 fat garlic clove, peeled
½ teaspoon ground cumin, plus extra to serve
3 tablespoons tahini
2–3 tablespoons lemon juice
100–150ml (3½–5fl oz) water
1 teaspoon black onion (nigella) seeds, to serve
salt and pepper

PER SERVING WITH CAULIFLOWER:
NET CARBS 3g | FIBRE 2g | PROTEIN 2g | FAT 9g | 98kcal

PER SERVING WITH CHICKPEAS:
NET CARBS 8g | FIBRE 4g | PROTEIN 4g | FAT 10g | 146kcal

Heat the oven to 220°C/200°C fan (425°F), Gas Mark 7. Line a baking tray with baking paper.

Lay the cauliflower on the lined baking tray. Drizzle over 2 tablespoons of the oil and season with salt and pepper. Toss the cauliflower to make sure all of the florets have some oil and seasoning.

Roast in the oven for 20–25 minutes until the cauliflower is lightly browned and softened. Remove from the oven and slide the paper off the tray to a cold work surface to cool.

Once the cauliflower is at room temperature, put it into a blender along with the remaining ingredients and blitz, adding enough water to obtain a smooth, soft consistency. Adjust the lemon juice and salt to taste. Transfer to a serving dish and top with a few black onion seeds, pepper, more cumin or just a dash of olive oil, as you like.

TAHINI DRESSING

This tangy, nutty dressing has a consistency like mayonnaise and is perfect dolloped on salads, roasted vegetables, hard-boiled eggs or with the za'atar flatbread on page 178.

Serves 6

200ml (7fl oz) 10% fat Greek yoghurt
3 tablespoons tahini
2 tablespoons extra-virgin olive oil
1 garlic clove, finely grated
2 tablespoons lemon juice, or more to taste
pinch of salt and pepper

PER SERVING:
NET CARBS 3g | FIBRE 1g | PROTEIN 3g | FAT 12g | 129kcal

Simply mix the ingredients together in a small bowl or jar and add 2–3 tablespoons of water to dilute the dressing to the desired consistency. Season to taste with extra lemon juice, salt and pepper if necessary to achieve a balance.

Use straight away or keep in the refrigerator for up to 3 days.

CUCUMBER RAITA

This is wonderfully cooling with any hot and spicy dish or with the za'atar flatbreads (see page 178). It will keep in the refrigerator for a couple of days. See the photo on page 69.

Always use whole, full-fat options of live yoghurt, as they usually contain only milk and healthy bacteria for your gut. They will leave you fuller for longer and taste way better than low-fat versions. I like to use kefir if I want a runny dressing and full-fat, thick Greek yoghurt for thick dips.

Serves 8

1 long cucumber (approx. 300g/10½oz), peeled and finely chopped
250g (9oz) 10% fat Greek yoghurt
1 heaped tablespoon finely chopped coriander leaves and stems
1 heaped tablespoon finely chopped mint leaves, plus a few, shredded, to serve
2–3 teaspoons ground cumin, to taste
hot green chilli (to taste), finely chopped, or a pinch of chilli flakes
salt
freshly ground black pepper, to serve

PER SERVING:
NET CARBS 2g | FIBRE 0g | PROTEIN 3g | FAT 4g | 53kcal

Mix the ingredients together and season to taste, adding more cumin or chilli to your liking. Season to taste with salt, then finish with a twist of black pepper and a few shredded mint leaves.

GREEN CHILLI AND HERB KEFIR DRESSING

I love live, natural kefir, so came up with this way of using it in a dressing. Either use the drinking kefir for a runny dressing or kefir yoghurt for a thicker sauce. It is wonderful over pretty much everything – hard-boiled eggs, barbecued meats or fish, or a simple green salad. If you make sure your kefir doesn't contain sugar or flavourings, you are good to go, happy in the knowledge your gut flora will love this as much as you do. Pictured on the left on page 73.

Serves 4 (makes 150g/5½oz)

25g (1oz) fresh mixed herbs (such as mint, dill, chives, parsley, chervil and celery leaves)
2 tablespoons extra-virgin olive oil
2 teaspoons lemon juice
½–1 green chilli, to taste
1 small garlic clove, peeled
pinch of salt
plenty of freshly ground black pepper
100g (3½oz) kefir drink or full-fat thick kefir or 10% fat Greek yoghurt

PER SERVING:
NET CARBS 1g | FIBRE 0g | PROTEIN 1g | FAT 8g | 77kcal

Make the sauce by whizzing the herbs, oil, lemon juice, chilli, garlic and seasoning and 50ml (2fl oz) of the kefir together in a small food-processor. Combine with the rest of the kefir. Alternatively, finely chop the herbs, chilli and garlic by hand and stir into the remaining ingredients. Season to taste and pour into a serving bowl. Store in the refrigerator until serving; it will keep for up to 4 days.

AVO NON-MAYO

This is from my friend Shirley Booth, who prefers to make this pale green, creamy alternative over having a standard, ultra-processed mayonnaise. It's packed with flavour, quick to whip together and goes with just about everything. Pictured centre, opposite.

Serves 8 (makes 225g/8oz)

100g (3½oz) avocado flesh (from about 1 medium avocado)
100g (3½oz) ricotta cheese
1–2 tablespoons lemon juice, plus extra to taste
finely grated zest of ¼–½ lemon, to taste
1 small garlic clove, peeled
2 tablespoons extra-virgin olive oil
3 tablespoons cold water
salt and pepper

PER SERVING:
NET CARBS 1g | FIBRE 1g | PROTEIN 1g | FAT 7g | 70kcal

Put all the ingredients in a small food processor and blend together, or simply grate the garlic and mash the ingredients together with a fork in a bowl. Taste and adjust the seasoning and lemon to your liking. Transfer to a serving bowl or a container and keep in the refrigerator for up to 4 days.

CHERMOULA

Did you know that 'herb' usually refers to the fresh leaves of a plant and 'spice' usually refers to the dried seeds or root of a plant? This zingy, flavour-packed Moroccan seasoning mix contains both fresh herbs and dried spices. Other versions include ginger, turmeric, coriander seed and plenty more, but this is our easy, fast and delicious blend. Use it sparingly over salmon, roast chicken, roasted vegetables or fried tofu. Pictured right, opposite.

Serves 6 (makes 100g/3½oz)

25g (1oz) coriander stems and leaves
15g (½oz) parsley stems and leaves
1–2 tablespoons lemon juice, plus extra to taste
1 small garlic clove, peeled
¼ teaspoon chilli flakes
¼ teaspoon salt, plus extra to taste
½ teaspoon paprika
½ teaspoon ground cumin
6 tablespoons extra-virgin olive oil

PER SERVING:
NET CARBS 0g | FIBRE 0g | PROTEIN 0g | FAT 14g | 121kcal

Put all the ingredients into a small food processor and blitz until you have a smooth paste. Taste and adjust to your liking with extra lemon juice, salt and chilli flakes.

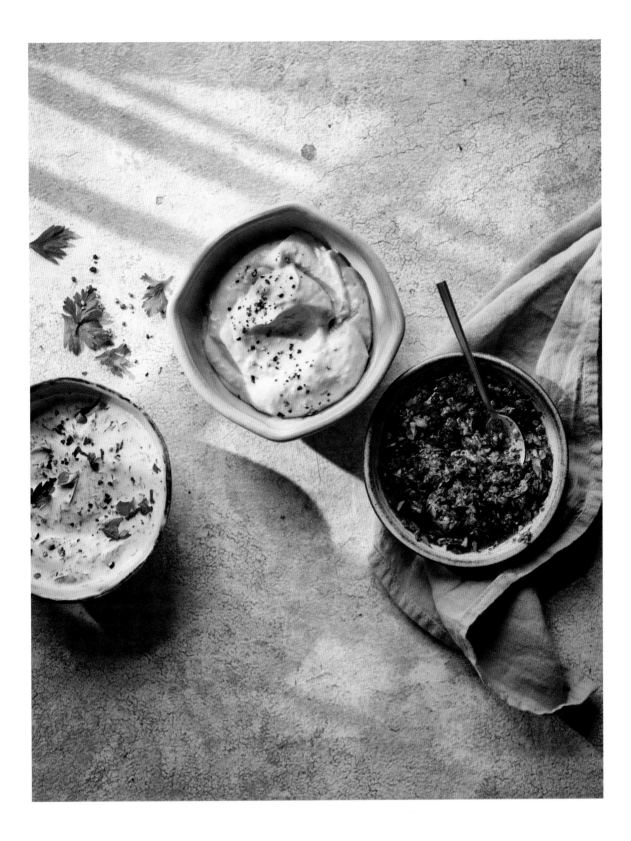

PROPER GRAVY

Serves 12
(makes approx. 600ml/20fl oz)

2 carrots, roughly chopped
2 onions, roughly chopped
2 celery sticks, roughly chopped
100g (3½oz) unsmoked bacon
    lardons or chopped streaky
    bacon rashers
2 bay leaves
2 sprigs of rosemary or sage
8 chicken wings
2 tablespoons extra-virgin olive oil
2 litres (3½ pints) just-boiled
    water
250ml (9fl oz) dry white wine
2 tablespoons cornflour (optional)
salt and pepper

PER 50ML (2FL OZ) SERVING:
NET CARBS 2g | FIBRE 0g
PROTEIN 0g | FAT 2g | 41kcal

A delicious gravy that can be made ahead of time. One thing I have realized over the years is that any leftover gravy makes a homemade soup come alive, so do freeze any for a soup day.

Heat the oven to 200°C/180°C fan (400°F), Gas Mark 6.

Put the vegetables into a roasting dish (that is suitable to heat on the hob later) and scatter over the bacon and herbs. Lay the chicken wings over the top to protect the vegetables from burning and drizzle over the oil. Season lightly with salt and pepper.

Cook in the oven for 1½ hours or until the chicken is roasted to a golden brown but not burned. Remove the tray from the oven and transfer the chicken and vegetables to a large saucepan. Put the dish over a medium-high heat on the hob and add the wine. Let it bubble and dissolve any brown sticky areas from the tray. When the wine has reduced by half tip it into the saucepan along with any remaining brown bits scraped from the dish.

Add the hot water and bring to the boil. Reduce the heat to a gentle boil and simmer for 2 hours or until it has reduced by half.

Use a potato masher to break up the chicken and crush the vegetables. Strain the stock into a bowl through a sieve, squeezing out as much flavour as possible from the chicken and vegetables with a wooden spoon.

Pour the liquid back into a saucepan and season to taste. If you prefer the gravy thicker, mix the cornflour with a splash of water in a bowl and add this to the gravy over the heat. Stir until thickened. The gravy is now ready to use – chill and store in the refrigerator for 3 days or freeze for up to 3 months.

'BREAD' SAUCE

This was always one of my favourite parts of Christmas lunch, but when we all became low-carb, it seemed pointless to make it. Now that I have discovered the joys of cauliflower, I realize I can make it into 'bread' sauce. I am happy to say it is a hit with the whole family and is back on our festive table again. Almond milk is lower in carbs than cows' milk, but either works.

Serves 8

1 small onion, halved
8 cloves
200g (7oz) cauliflower, riced (see page 156)
150ml (5fl oz) full-fat almond or cows' milk
50ml (2fl oz) double cream
1 bay leaf
10g (¼oz) butter
salt and pepper

PER SERVING:
NET CARBS 2g | FIBRE 0g | PROTEIN 1g | FAT 4g | 42kcal

Stud half the onion with the cloves, so they offer their flavour but don't become lost in the sauce. Put all the ingredients together in a medium saucepan and bring to the boil. Reduce the heat and gently simmer for 20–30 minutes or until the sauce has thickened, stirring occasionally to break up the cauliflower.

Adjust the seasoning, then pick out the bay leaf and onion. Serve straight away or cool the sauce and keep in the refrigerator for up to 5 days.

CRANBERRY SAUCE

Cranberries are naturally sour in flavour. If you are a hardened no-sugar person, you may find the sweetness of the orange is enough for you. Others may prefer minimal honey or erythritol. This sauce keeps in the refrigerator for up to a week or can be frozen.

Serves 8

300g (10½oz) cranberries
3 long peelings of pared orange zest, plus juice of 1 orange
1 tablespoon honey or 2 tablespoons erythritol, or more to taste
100ml (3½fl oz) dry white wine

PER SERVING WITH HONEY:
NET CARBS 6g | FIBRE 1g | PROTEIN 0g | FAT 0g | 39kcal

PER SERVING WITH ERYTHRITOL:
NET CARBS 4g | FIBRE 1g | PROTEIN 0g | FAT 0g | 31kcal

Put all the ingredients into a saucepan and bring to the boil. Reduce the heat so that the mixture gently bubbles and continue to cook, stirring frequently, for about 10 minutes until the berries begin to burst. At this point taste the sauce for sweetness and adjust accordingly. Remove from the heat and leave to cool before serving.

LOW-CARB SWAP

COOKED PASTA RIBBONS

(200G/7OZ)

47G CARBS

VS

BUTTERED CABBAGE RIBBONS (PAGE 107)

(200G/7OZ)

7G CARBS

This chapter will teach you simple and efficient cooking skills for tasty meals within 30 minutes. From great ways to cook seabass and white fish fillets, to how to butterfly a chicken, make Smash Burgers, cook the perfect omelette and plenty more.

Since I have disposed of our non-stick frying pans and replaced them with stainless steel frying pans that should last a lifetime, I have been using our chef Mattia Barbieri's tip from when he was learning to cook. The tip is to place a piece of baking paper in the bottom of the frying pan, which allows you to cook delicate fish or skinless chicken without worrying that it will stick and tear. I love it! Cooking is so much more relaxing if you have less that can go wrong!

I have also given plenty of suggestions for what to have instead of pasta. If you are cooking for the family, make the same sauce for everyone but while the kids eat pasta you can have vegetable alternatives made from leeks, courgettes or cabbage to avoid the glucose spikes.

QUICK
& EASY

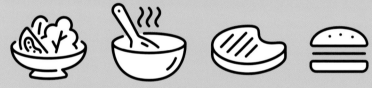

TOMATO AND PEPPER SOUP

Serves 4

3 tablespoons extra-virgin olive oil, plus a drizzle to serve

1 large red pepper, cored, deseeded and roughly chopped

1 white onion or small leek, finely chopped

1 large celery stick, roughly chopped

1 fat garlic clove, peeled and lightly crushed

a little red chilli (to taste), finely chopped, or a pinch of chilli flakes

1 teaspoon salt

400g (14oz) can Italian plum tomatoes

600ml (20fl oz) vegetable or chicken stock or hot water

handful of parsley, leaves and stalks, finely chopped, or basil leaves, to serve

freshly ground black pepper

Optional additions

250g (9oz) Quick Fried Garlicky Prawns (see page 80)

4 tablespoons crème fraîche or 10% fat Greek yoghurt

1 teaspoon finely grated lemon zest

25g (1oz) Parmesan cheese

PER SERVING WITHOUT ADDITIONS:
NET CARBS 6g | FIBRE 3g | PROTEIN 1g | FAT 10g | 126kcal

This popular comfort food is easy to make at home. This is a lovely, light starter soup. Make it into a main course by adding protein in the form of a couple of poached eggs or a big spoonful of goats' cheese or leftover cooked chicken. However, our favourite way to serve this is topped with the Quick Fried Garlicky Prawns on page 80 and a swirl of vodka! It makes a great talking point as a starter for a party and tastes a little like a Bloody Mary.

Heat the oil for 2 minutes in a medium saucepan over a medium–high heat. Add the pepper, onion or leek, celery, garlic, chilli, salt and pepper, turn down the heat to medium and cook for around 15 minutes, or until everything has lost its crunch.

Add the tomatoes, stock or water and bring to the boil. Turn down the heat to lower it to a gentle boil and continue to cook for 15 minutes, breaking up the tomatoes with a wooden spoon or spatula.

Blend the soup with a stick blender or leave it chunky if you prefer. Taste and add more seasoning as needed.

Serve the soup in warm bowls with a swirl of your best olive oil and a scattering of the herbs or add one of the additions listed on the left.

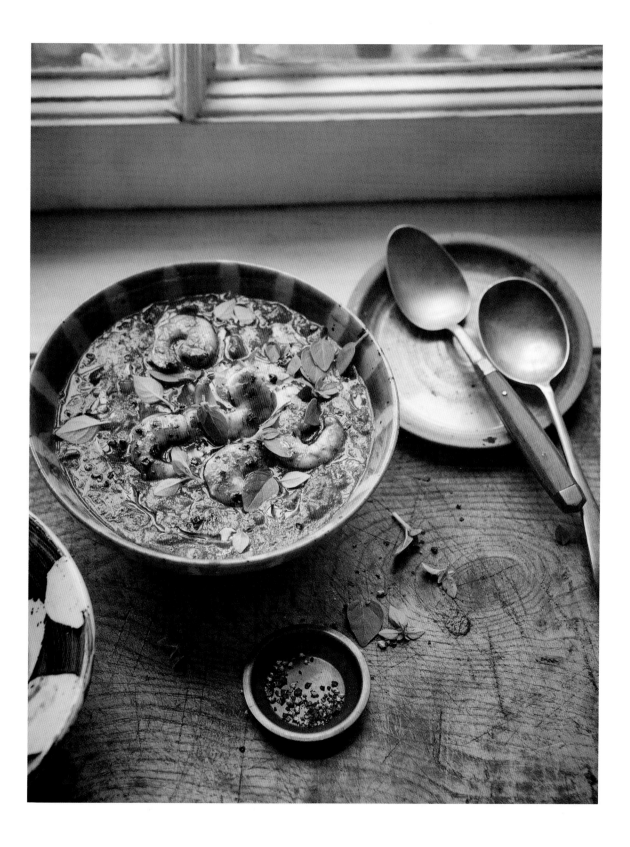

QUICK FRIED GARLICKY PRAWNS

This is a really quick stir-fried recipe for spicy prawns to eat with low-carb bread or Spanish tapas-style, or to add to the Tomato and Pepper Soup on page 78. Use frozen or fresh prawns depending on your budget, but if possible get ones with the heads on (and leave them on to cook) as that is where the flavour lies. Fresh ones need peeling, and black veins should be removed from their spines.

Serves 2

1 tablespoon extra-virgin olive oil
1 fat garlic clove, crushed or finely chopped
a little fresh red chilli (to taste), finely chopped, or a pinch of chilli flakes
250g (9oz) raw prawns, peeled and heads left on if possible
handful of parsley, leaves and stalks finely chopped
salt and pepper

PER SERVING:
NET CARBS 0g | FIBRE 0g | PROTEIN 30g | FAT 7g | 183kcal

Heat the oil in a medium frying pan over a medium–high heat. When hot, add the garlic and chilli and fry for 2 minutes, then add the prawns and season with salt and plenty of pepper. Continue to fry, tossing the prawns in the pan as they cook, for 5 minutes, until they are completely pink.

Taste and adjust the seasoning as necessary. Serve straight away with tomato soup or some low-carb bread.

SPICY MACKEREL PÂTÉ

This takes minutes to whip up from store-cupboard ingredients and yet makes a satisfying lunch at home or at work. I was going to use cans of ready-flavoured spicy mackerel until I realized they contained 5g (1/8oz) carbs per 100g (3½oz), compared to 0g carbs in the plain mackerel in oil, so beware – sugar gets everywhere!

Serves 2 as a main course or 6 as a dip

2 cans (approx. 160g/5¾oz total drained weight) mackerel in olive oil or water
1 tablespoon extra-virgin olive oil (if using mackerel in water)
50g (1¾oz) 10% fat Greek yoghurt
1 garlic clove, grated
¼ teaspoon salt
plenty of freshly ground black pepper, plus extra to serve
pinch chilli powder, plus extra to taste
finely grated zest and juice of ½ small lemon

To serve

6 small lettuce leaves or 2 slices of low-carb bread
2 celery sticks, finely chopped, plus leaves
½ lemon, cut into wedges

PER SERVING FOR 2 ON LETTUCE:
NET CARBS 3g | FIBRE 1g | PROTEIN 21g | FAT 14g, 228kcal

Drain most of the oil (if it is olive) from the mackerel, leaving a tablespoon; if it's water, drain it all and add the tablespoon of extra-virgin olive oil. Flake the fish into a mixing bowl and stir in the remaining ingredients. Taste and add more seasoning or chilli.

Pile the pâté on the lettuce leaves or bread. Top with the celery, leaves and a few twists of pepper and serve with wedges of lemon.

CHIVE AND SMOKED CHEDDAR OMELETTE

Serves 1

3 medium eggs
small handful of herbs (such as chives, dill, flat-leaf parsley or coriander), finely chopped
¼ teaspoon fine salt
2 teaspoons ghee, butter or extra-virgin olive oil
20g (¾oz) smoked or mature Cheddar cheese, grated
freshly ground black pepper

Optional additions
50g (1¾oz) cooked ham, bacon or chicken, roughly chopped
a few drops of hot sauce or a pinch of chilli flakes

PER CHEESE OMELETTE: NET CARBS 2g FIBRE 0g | PROTEIN 21g FAT 29g, 356kcal

PER OMELETTE WITH HAM: NET CARBS 3g | FIBRE 0g | PROTEIN 38g FAT 46g | 590kcal

For a while the humble omelette was often forgotten in our house. But since our son Flavio has been living in Paris we have been reminded of the French passion for omelettes, so now eat this simple delight at least once a week and wonder what on earth we did without them. Omelettes are the perfect low-carb meal, ready in 5 to 10 minutes, and lend themselves perfectly to using up leftovers. I find a 3-egg omelette makes a satisfying meal for one. Alternatively, share this amount and add a salad or some low-carb bread.

Make sure you have a warm plate ready and everything you need to hand to work quickly.

Crack the eggs into a bowl, add the herbs, plenty of black pepper and the salt and whisk with a fork until you can't see the yolk from the white.

Melt the ghee, butter or oil in a non-stick frying pan over a medium heat. Swirl it around to coat the base of the pan. Increase the heat to medium–high and add the eggs. Use a spatula to move the eggs around for about a minute, criss-crossing the pan to get the runny eggs to the bottom, but making sure there are no holes in the omelette. When the outer edges become opaque, run the spatula around the rim of the pan to loosen it. Shake the pan to make sure the omelette can slide.

Scatter the cheese, and any other additions, over the half furthest away from the handle. Now use the spatula to loosen the edge nearest the handle and tip the pan to help curl it towards the half with the stuffing. Cook the omelette for 2 minutes more, or until the eggs are cooked to your liking; they should be a little wet inside.

Now switch hands so that you can tip the omelette on to a serving plate – this action will fold the bottom over the top. It should be a neat, rolled omelette. If it all goes horribly wrong, just call it scrambled eggs and have another go another day! It took me several attempts to perfect an omelette, but you can see how to do it on our website (see page 205).

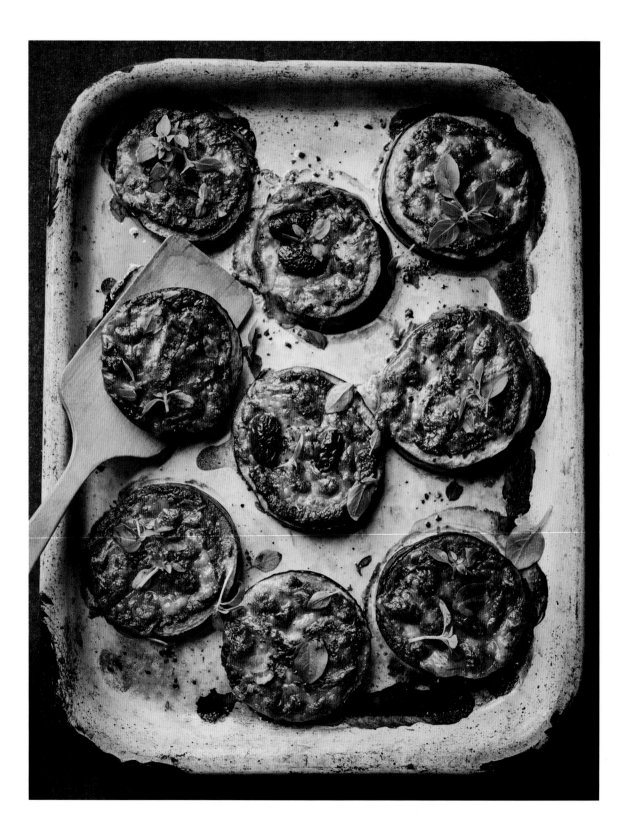

PIZZA AUBERGINES

Serves 2

3 tablespoons extra-virgin olive oil
1 large aubergine (approx.
    300g/10½oz)
1 heaped tablespoon tomato
    purée
½ teaspoon dried oregano
125g (4½oz) mozzarella cheese,
    roughly torn and drained
handful of basil leaves
salt and pepper

Additional toppings (optional)
pitted black olives
anchovies
tuna
slices of salami

**PER SERVING WITH NO ADDITIONAL
TOPPINGS:** NET CARBS 6g | FIBRE 5g
PROTEIN 15g | FAT 36g | 418kcal

Aubergines make the perfect low-carb pizza base. Served with a green salad, this an easy lunch or supper that can be made in 30 minutes. Alternatively, serve them as individual canapés. The possibilities for toppings are endless, such as feta or halloumi instead of mozzarella, or a smoked cheese; we love smoked scamorza. Bump up the protein content by adding tuna, sardines, leftover chicken, salami or crumbled sausage over them before grilling.

Heat the oven to 220°C/200°C (425°F), Gas Mark 7. Brush a baking tray with a little of the olive oil.

Cut the top off the aubergine and then slice it into 1cm- (½-inch-) thick circles. You should have around 10 slices depending on the size of your aubergine. Lay them down on the lined tray and brush the tops only with the remaining olive oil. Lightly season. Bake them in the oven for 17–20 minutes, until lightly browned and soft to the touch.

Meanwhile, mix the tomato purée with the oregano and season, adding 1–2 tablespoons of water to dilute it into a sauce.

Remove the aubergines from the oven and heat the grill to hot.

Spread the tomato sauce over each slice of aubergine with the back of a spoon, leaving a narrow border around the edges. Top each slice with the torn mozzarella and any additional toppings you like.

Put the tray under the grill and cook for another 6–8 minutes, or until the cheese is bubbling and starting to brown. Remove from the oven and serve scattered with the basil.

SPICY ROOT PATTIES

Serves 4 (makes 12 patties)

For the patties

450g (1lb) trimmed and peeled
root vegetables (such as swede,
carrot, parsnip, celeriac and
turnip)

100g (3½oz) trimmed leek,
cleaned and finely chopped

2 eggs

250g (9oz) halloumi cheese,
coarsely grated

60g (2¼oz) chickpea flour

15g (½oz) chives, parsley or
coriander, finely chopped

2 teaspoons ground cumin

2 teaspoons chilli flakes or finely
chopped fresh hot chilli

Optional additions

4 fried eggs

handful of coriander or parsley

PER SERVING WITHOUT EGG:
NET CARBS 19g | FIBRE 5g
PROTEIN 24g | FAT 20g | 361kcal

These are a great supper dish and can be made in batches and kept chilled in the refrigerator for up to 4 days, or frozen for 3 months. We love them with a fried egg on top, or with boiled eggs if we take them for a packed lunch, for extra protein. The halloumi is salty enough that you don't need to add any further seasoning.

Line a baking tray with baking paper. Fill a kettle and put it on.

Coarsely grate the root vegetables in a food processor or by hand. Put them into a bowl and pour over enough boiling water to cover. Leave to stand for 2 minutes, stirring a couple of times. Pour the vegetables into a colander and leave to drain for a few minutes. When cool enough to touch, thoroughly squeeze the mixture in a tea towel to get rid of the excess water. Drop the squeezed vegetables into a large mixing bowl.

Heat the oven to 220°C/200°C fan (425°F), Gas Mark 7.

Now add the leek, eggs, halloumi, flour, herbs and spices and stir through to combine. Divide the mixture into 12 (each roughly 70g/2½oz) balls and gently squeeze them into burger shapes with your hands, squeezing out any further moisture. Lay each one on the prepared baking tray and flatten slightly, then bake in the oven for 20–25 minutes until golden brown and just firm to the touch.

Serve with a fried egg on top if you like, scattered with coriander or parsley, if using.

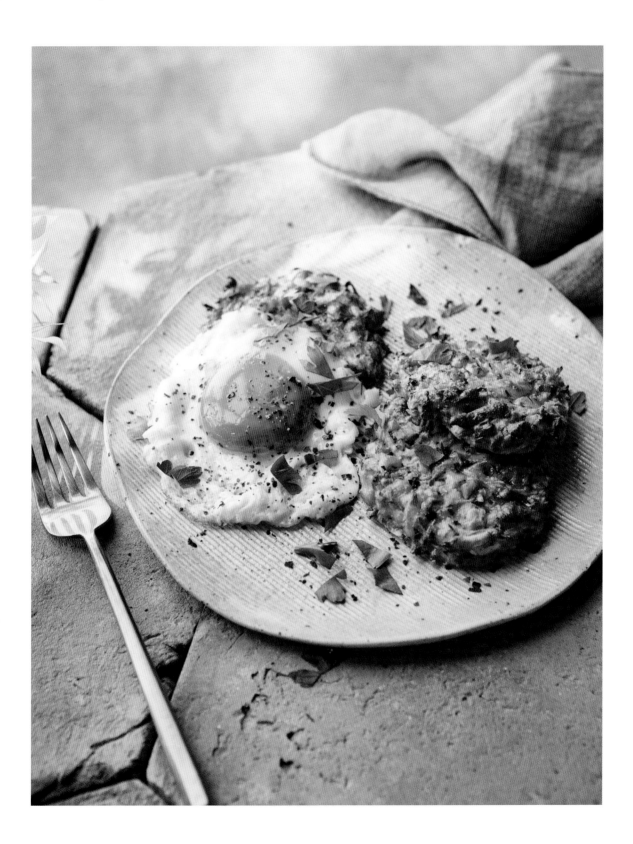

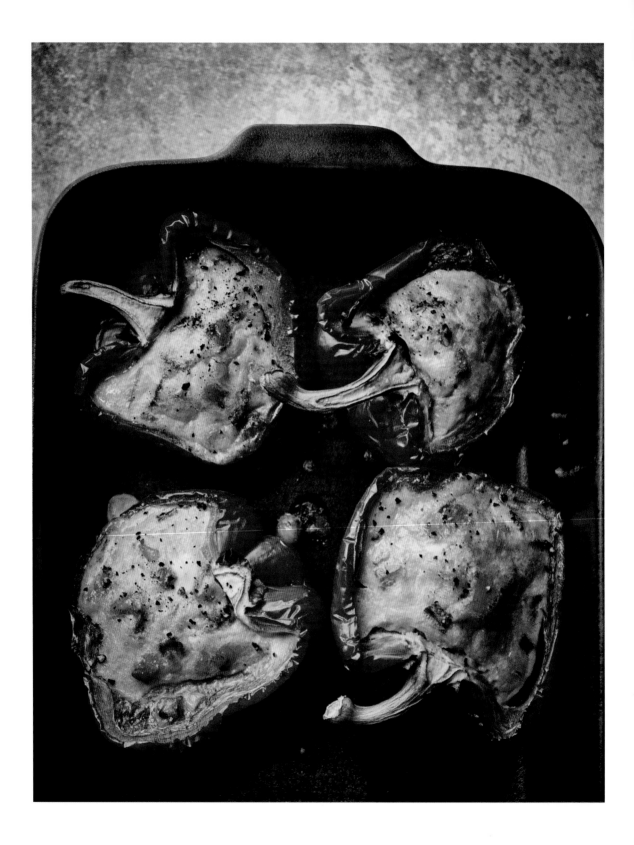

PEPPER QUICHES

Serves 2

2 red peppers, halved, cored and deseeded
1 tablespoon extra-virgin olive oil
1 small onion or fat spring onion, finely chopped
100g (3½oz) smoked bacon or ham, diced, or 1 sausage, peeled and crumbled
4 eggs
25g (1oz) mature Cheddar or other hard cheese, grated
salt and pepper

PER SERVING OF 2 HALVES:
NET CARBS 11g | FIBRE 4g | PROTEIN 32g
FAT 38g | 536kcal

Pepper halves are brilliant, colourful vessels for a variety of fillings and cook perfectly in half an hour. I have used the typical flavours of French quiche Lorraine, but you could use up whatever is in your refrigerator, such as leftover roast vegetables and various cheeses, or a handful of chickpeas or cannellini beans instead of the bacon.

Heat the oven to 220°C/200°C fan (425°F), Gas Mark 7.

Put the peppers in a small, oven dish or roasting tray. They should fit snugly so that they support one another and can be easily filled. Roast them in the oven for 10 minutes, then remove and set aside.

Meanwhile, make the filling by heating the oil in a medium frying pan and gently frying the onions and bacon, ham or sausage together over a medium heat for 5–7 minutes until the onions are translucent and the meat is lightly browned. When done, tip the contents of the frying pan on a plate to cool.

Beat the eggs in a mixing bowl with a good pinch of salt and plenty of pepper. Stir in the cheese and then add the onion and bacon mixture. Pour this mixture into the peppers, making sure they can't tip over.
If any halves worry you, support them with a little scrunched-up foil.

Cook for 20 minutes, or until the peppers are tender and the filling is set and lightly browned.

Serve with a salad or some green vegetables.

COBB SALAD

Serves 4

For the vinaigrette

1 tablespoon red wine vinegar or
    cider vinegar
2 teaspoons lemon juice
4 tablespoons extra-virgin olive
    oil
1 teaspoon Dijon mustard
¼ teaspoon salt
plenty of freshly ground black
    pepper
1 small garlic clove, grated
    (optional)

For the salad

4 eggs
2 tablespoons extra-virgin olive oil
4 smoked bacon rashers, roughly
    chopped
200g (7oz) chicken breast or
    breast fillets, or leftover roast
    chicken or turkey
1 romaine heart or the equivalent
    in other salad leaves, torn or
    shredded into bite-sized pieces
12 cherry or round tomatoes,
    halved or sliced
100g (3½oz) feta, blue or other
    crumbly cheese
1 avocado, sliced
salt and pepper
handful of parsley leaves

PER SERVING: NET CARBS 10g | FIBRE 6g
PROTEIN 30g | FAT 41g | 544kcal

I have always loved the neat rows of colourful ingredients, waiting to be enjoyed in various combinations, in this American chopped salad. Named after Robert Cobb who owned the Brown Derby restaurant in Hollywood, this salad has been going strong since the 1930s.

The protein comes from the chicken, bacon and eggs, so it's filling as well as tasty. Take leftovers to work in a jar with the dressing at the bottom of the jar, then the chicken, and then the leaves on top so they don't become soggy. A butterflied chicken breast cooks quickly, so if you are not already familiar with it, butterflying is an ideal skill to learn.

Shake all the vinaigrette ingredients together in a jar until emulsified. Set aside.

Bring a small pot of water to the boil. Gently lower in the eggs and boil for 8 minutes. Remove from the heat and drain, then run cold water over the eggs to quickly chill them. Break the shell of each egg; this will ensure they don't develop a blue ring inside. Shell them once cool.

Heat the oil in a large frying pan over a medium heat. Add the bacon and cook for around 8 minutes, or until crispy on both sides. Transfer to a plate to cool, keeping the juices in the pan. Once cool enough, coarsely chop the bacon and set aside.

To butterfly the chicken, lay a breast on a chopping board with the pointed end facing you. Starting at the top, use a sharp knife to cut into the side while holding the top flat with your other hand. Cut almost through to the other side as if cutting into a book while keeping the spine intact. Now open out the chicken to resemble a butterfly. Repeat with the other breast(s). Cover them with baking paper then use a meat mallet or rolling pin to evenly flatten the meat until it is around 1cm (½ inch) thick. Remove the paper. Scatter over the seasoning. Leave the chicken on the board and thoroughly wash your hands.

Reheat the pan with the bacon juices over a medium–high heat, adding a little more oil if there isn't much left. Use a fork to transfer the chicken to the pan, and cook for 4 minutes on each side until well browned and cooked through. Transfer the chicken to a clean chopping board and cut through the thickest part to ensure it isn't pink inside.

Once the chicken is cool enough to handle, slice it into bite-sized pieces. Cut the eggs in half. Evenly spread the lettuce over a large plate, then arrange the chicken, bacon, tomatoes, cheese, eggs and avocado in rows on top. Sprinkle over the parsley and drizzle over half the dressing; serve the rest on the side in a jug.

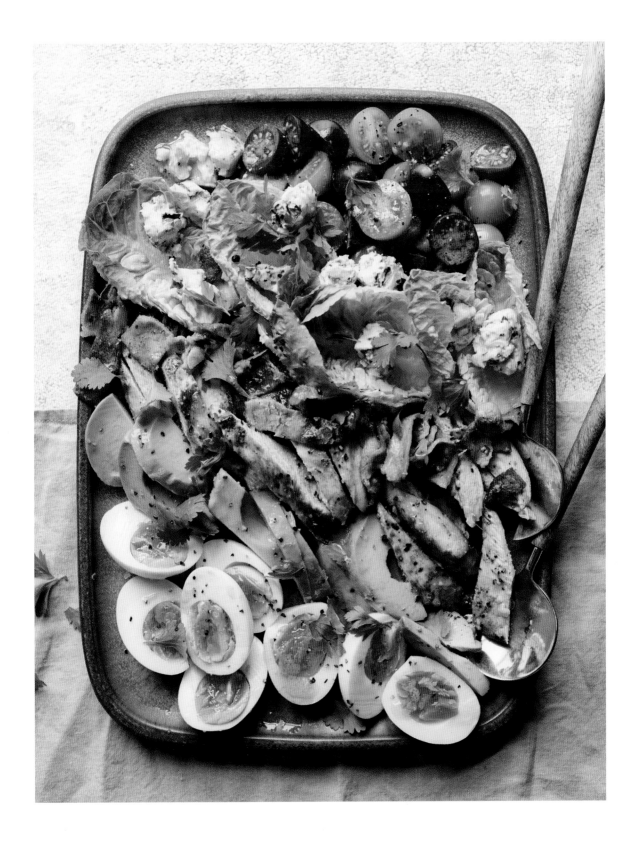

PAN-FRIED HALIBUT WITH BUTTER SAUCE

Serves 2

2 halibut, cod or other white fish
fillets, approx. 150g (5½oz) each
2 teaspoons extra-virgin olive oil
25g (1oz) butter
2 sprigs each of rosemary, sage
and thyme
2 teaspoons lemon juice or
2 tablespoons white wine
salt and pepper

PER SERVING: NET CARBS 0g | FIBRE 0g
PROTEIN 23g | FAT 18g | 249kcal

Head Chef Mattia Barbieri from our restaurant Caldesi in Marylebone, London, showed me this trick using baking paper for cooking fish that he was taught when he was learning to cook. I love the simple flavours of the herbs in the sauce, but this is also delicious with no herbs, or just one variety. Adding a little acidity in the form of lemon juice or white wine cuts through the butter and emulsifies it into a sauce. To finish, you could also add a splash of cream or a few capers, or garnish with some fresh parsley instead of using woody herbs in the sauce. Before you start, have everything ready around you, including your side dish.

Cut a piece of baking paper big enough to fit two fish fillets in a medium-sized frying pan. Season the fish all over, using your fingers to evenly spread it out.

Heat the frying pan over a high heat. Using tongs, lay the paper down on the surface of the hot pan. Add the oil and as soon as it has spread, lay the fish on top. Leave it to cook – it should be sizzling – for around 3 minutes, or until it has lightly browned underneath and has started to become opaque around the edges.

Use a spatula or fish slice to turn the fillets; to help, you can hold the fish on the top side with your fingers, as it will still be cold. Now leave the fillets to cook for around 2 minutes or until lightly browned underneath.

Add the butter and herbs. When the butter has melted and is foaming, tilt the pan and use a spoon to drizzle the herb butter over the fish. To check if the fish is done, feel the top of the fish; they should feel firm. You can also use a thermometer; they should be around 60°C (140°F) inside. If not, put the lid on and leave them to cook for a further 2 minutes.

Add the lemon juice or white wine and let it sizzle and evaporate for a couple of minutes. Serve the fish straight away or leave it to rest, off the heat, for up to 5 minutes. This is lovely with either of the mashes on pages 168–169 and green vegetables.

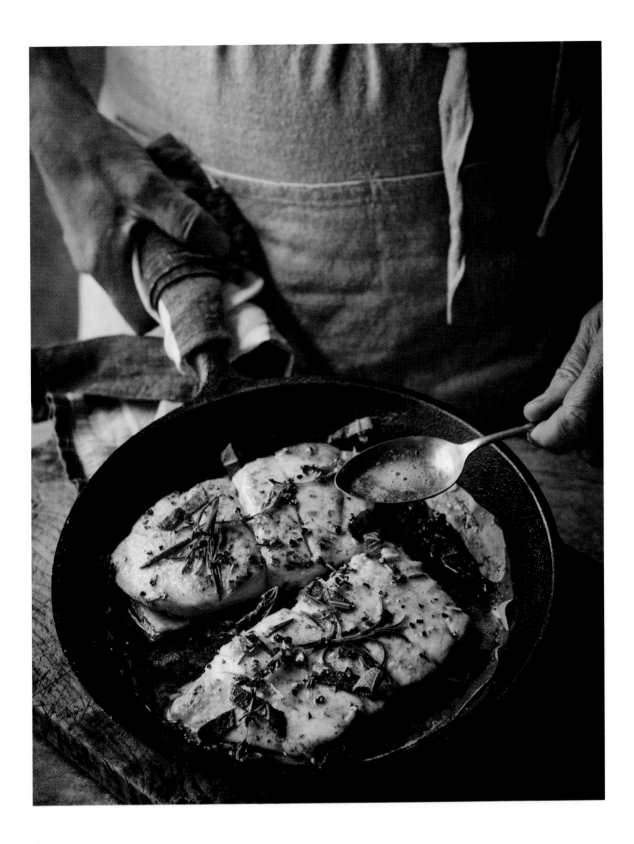

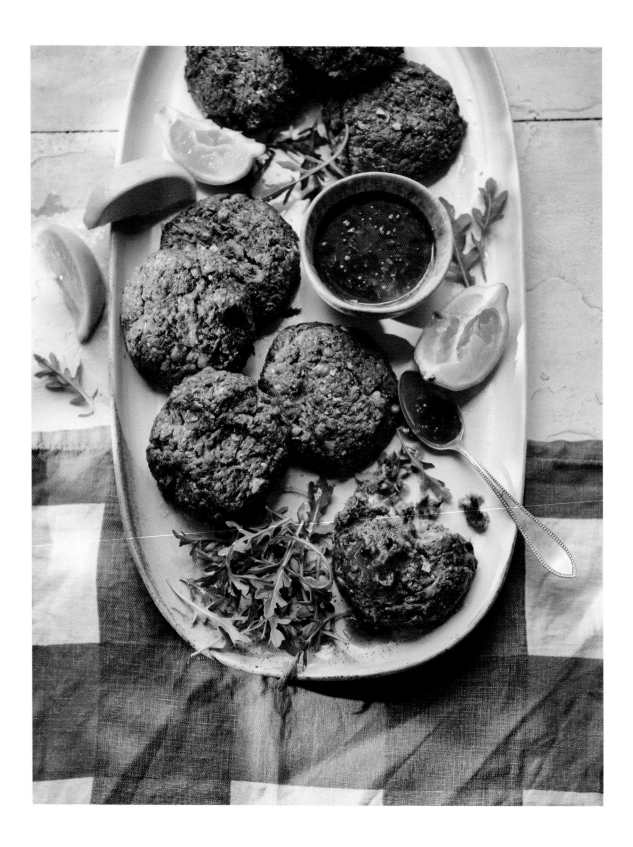

CURRIED FISHCAKES
WITH SPICY DIPPING SAUCE

Makes 8 medium or 20 small fishcakes

For the fishcakes
400g (14oz) can pilchards in tomato sauce
1 teaspoon salt
plenty of freshly ground black pepper
200g (7oz) cauliflower, riced (see page 156)
240g (8½oz) cooked and drained chickpeas
2 eggs
1 heaped tablespoon curry powder

For the dipping sauce
½–1 teaspoon chilli flakes, to taste
1 garlic clove, grated
1 heaped teaspoon finely grated fresh root ginger

lemon wedges, to serve

PER FISHCAKE, IF MAKING 8:
NET CARBS 8.8g | FIBRE 3g
PROTEIN 11g | FAT 6g | 131kcal

PER FISHCAKE, IF MAKING 20:
NET CARBS 4g | FIBRE 1g
PROTEIN 4g | FAT 2g | 52kcal

My family used to be a bit sniffy about canned pilchards, but they are a delicious and inexpensive source of protein, not to mention omega-3 and vitamins. These are based on a Sri Lankan recipe a friend showed me, and now I am a convert. I've used the tomato sauce from the pilchards as a dip, so that the whole can is used. These fishcakes can be served as a main course with salad or made half the size and served as nibbles. Use canned or freshly cooked chickpeas.

Heat the oven to 200°C/180°C fan (400°F), Gas Mark 6.

Drain the pilchards through a sieve over a saucepan to separate them from the tomato sauce. Set the pan aside.

Put the fish with the remaining fishcake ingredients into a bowl and use a fork to mash them together. Take a heaped teaspoon of the mixture and flatten it into a thin, miniature patty. Fry this in a little oil in a frying pan until crisp. Taste and decide if the mixture needs more seasoning or curry powder. When you are happy with the flavour, divide the mixture into 8 or 20 balls and shape them into patties. Put them on a baking tray and bake in the oven for 20 minutes, or until lightly browned.

To make the sauce, add the chilli flakes, garlic and ginger to the pan with the tomato sauce and place over a low heat for 5 minutes until warmed through. Taste and adjust the chilli heat accordingly. Pour into a serving bowl.

Serve the fishcakes warm or at room temperature with the dipping sauce, lemon wegdes, and a salad, if you like.

SALMON AND ASPARAGUS TRAYBAKE

Serves 2

275g (9¾oz) asparagus and/or
  Mediterranean vegetables (such
  as onion, peppers or courgettes)
3 tablespoons extra-virgin olive oil
  or butter
4 tablespoons dry white wine or
  water
2 tablespoons small capers in salt
  or brine
2 salmon steaks (approx.
  130g/4½oz each)
1 lemon
salt and pepper

PER SERVING: NET CARBS 4g | FIBRE 3g
PROTEIN 37g | FAT 31g | 470kcal

Oily fish such as salmon are perfect for a ridiculously simple traybake like this, as the oils stop them from drying out in the oven. Alter the vegetables according to what you have in the refrigerator or what's in season. I like peppers and courgettes in summer and broccoli or cauliflower all year round. I prefer the small capers in salt for flavour, but they need a good rinse in a sieve and might still be too salty, so go easy when adding more salt to the fish. You could also leave the capers and lemon out of this and serve it with the Green Chilli and Herb Kefir Dressing, Chermoula or Romesco in the Sauces & Dips chapter (see pages 71, 72 and 67).

Heat the oven to 220°C/200°C fan (425°F), Gas Mark 7.

Bend the asparagus spears one by one; they will snap where the woody part meets the softer tip. Discard the woody ends and rinse the tips. If using other vegetables, cut them into finger-width strips or circles.

Spread the vegetables over a baking tray. Season the vegetables and drizzle over half the oil or dot over half the butter. Pour over the wine or water and put the tray into the oven to roast for 10 minutes.

Meanwhile, rinse the capers of their salt or brine; taste them for saltiness.

Remove the tray from the oven and add the salmon, skin-side down, on top of the veg.. Pour over the remaining oil or dot over the remaining butter and season the fish. Pare the zest of half the lemon over them. Scatter over the capers and place the tray in the oven. Cook for another 10–12 minutes, or until the vegetables are cooked through and starting to brown, and the salmon fillets are firm rather than wobbly. You can also measure the temperature with a thermometer; the fish should be 63°C (145°F) inside the thickest point. If not, remove the vegetables or the fish if either is done, and continue to cook until both are ready.

Remove from the oven and serve with the ungrated half of the lemon, cut into wedges.

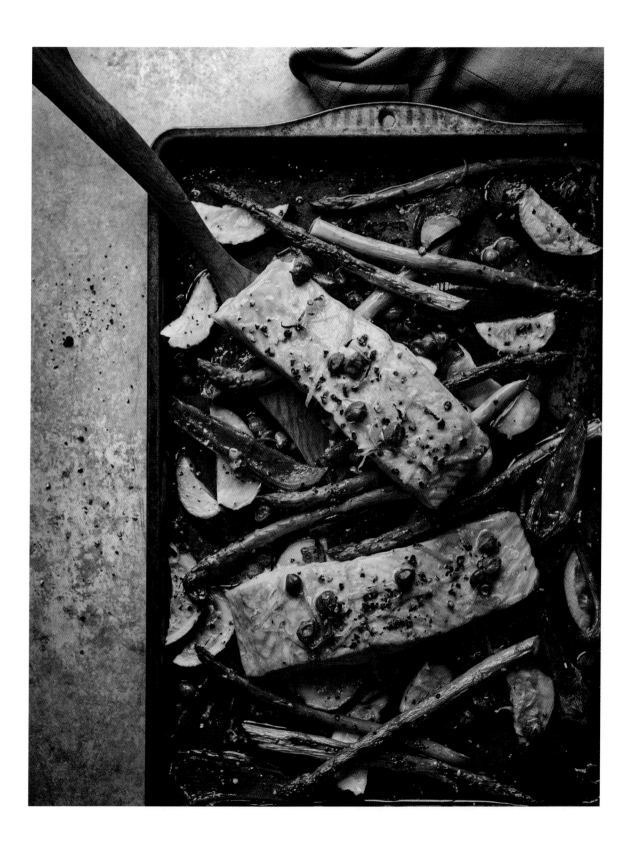

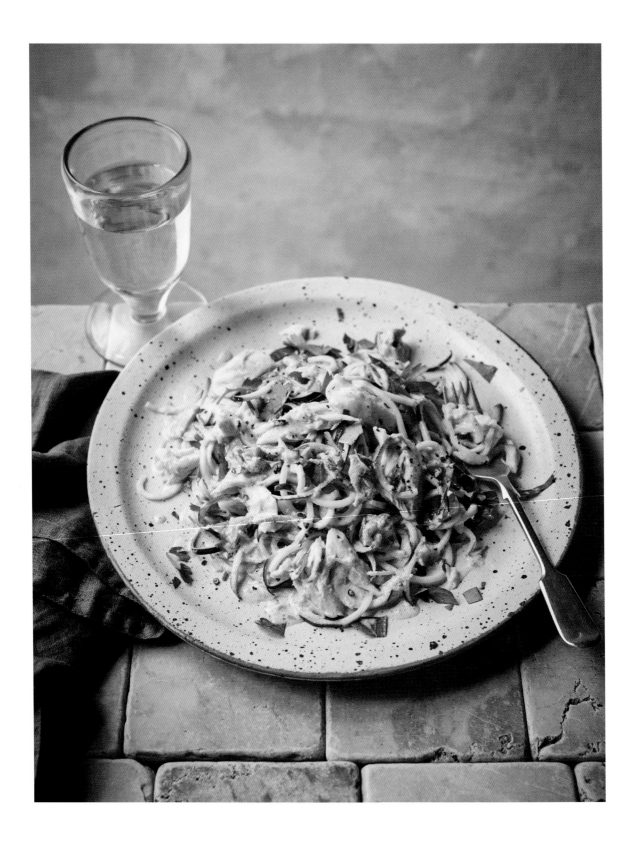

OVEN-BAKED SEABASS FILLETS WITH A LEMON CREAM SAUCE

Serves 2

2 seabass fillets (approx. 220g/
7¾oz total weight)
1 tablespoon extra-virgin olive oil
salt and pepper
2 portions courgetti (see page
107), to serve (optional)

For the sauce
25g (1oz) unsalted butter
1 garlic clove, crushed
¼ teaspoon chilli flakes or finely
chopped fresh hot chilli
(optional)
1 tomato, cut into 1cm (½-inch) dice
1 teaspoon finely grated lemon
zest, or more to taste
2 teaspoons lemon juice, or more
to taste
3 tablespoons crème fraîche or
double cream
2 tablespoons roughly chopped
flat-leaf parsley

PER SERVING OF ROASTED SEABASS:
NET CARBS 0g | FIBRE 0g | PROTEIN 19g
FAT 19g | 251kcal

PER SERVING WITH SAUCE:
NET CARBS 3g | FIBRE 1g | PROTEIN 20g
FAT 37g | 427kcal

**PER SERVING WITH SAUCE AND
COURGETTI:** NET CARBS 7g | FIBRE 3g
PROTEIN 23g | FAT 51g | 580kcal

This is a very easy, hands-free way to cook fillets of fish in the oven. Simply coated in olive oil and seasoning, the fish cooks in minutes and can be served whole or broken into a courgetti pasta sauce.

Here I have paired it with a lemony, creamy sauce, but it is also great with the Chermoula sauce (see page 72), the Green Chilli and Herb Kefir Dressing (see page 71) or the Herb Butter made with tarragon (see page 66).

Heat the oven to 220°C/200°C fan (425°F), Gas Mark 7. Line a baking tray with baking paper.

Lay the seabass skin-side down on the lined baking tray. Use your fingers to oil the surface of the fish. While you are doing this, feel for any bones, and remove with tweezers if you find any. Season evenly with salt and pepper. Cook for 10–15 minutes, or until cooked through and firm to the touch.

Make the sauce by heating the butter in a large frying pan. When it has melted, add the garlic, chilli, if using, and some salt and pepper, then cook for 2 minutes. Add the tomato, lemon zest and lemon juice. Reduce the heat, cook for 2 minutes and then add the crème fraîche or double cream and stir through as it warms. Taste the sauce and adjust the seasoning or lemon as necessary.

If you are keeping the fillets whole – remove the fish from the oven and carefully pour any juices from the tray into the sauce. Use a spatula or fish slice to transfer the fish to warm serving plates. Pour over the sauce and scatter over the parsley. Serve with green vegetables.

If you are serving with courgetti – remove the fish from the oven and pour any juices from the tray into the sauce. Use a spatula or fish slice to separate the fish from its skin (it should slide off). Break up the fish and transfer it to the sauce. Gently stir it into the sauce and serve over bowls of just-cooked courgetti, scattered with the parsley.

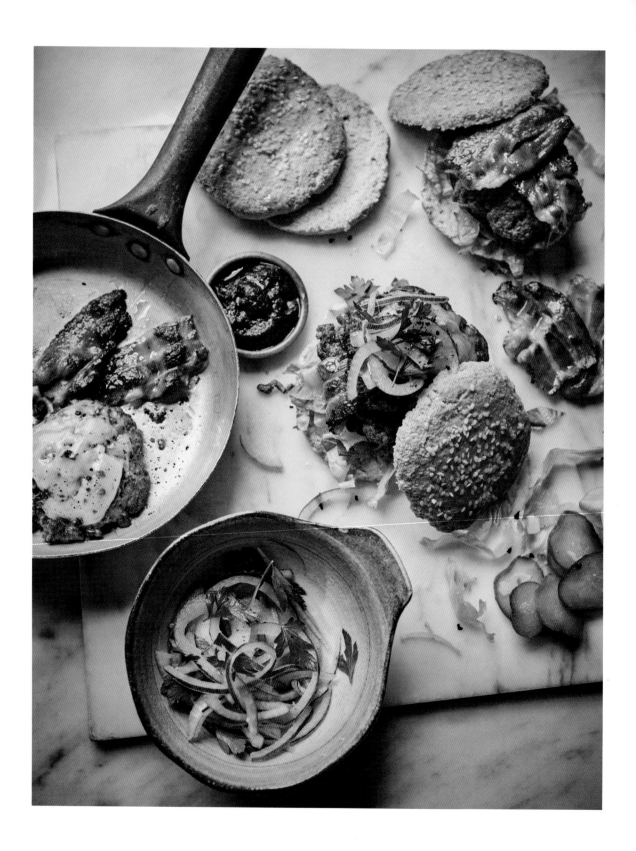

SMASH BACON CHEESE BURGERS

Serves 2

2 Sliders (see page 175)
2 teaspoons lard, chicken fat or
  dripping or ghee
4 streaky bacon rashers (approx.
  100g/3½oz), halved
250g (9oz) 15–20%-fat beef or
  lamb mince, either fresh or
  defrosted
½ teaspoon salt
plenty of freshly ground black
  pepper
20g (¾oz) mature or smoked
  Cheddar cheese, shaved
green salad, to serve (optional)

For the tomato sauce
1 tablespoon tomato purée
pinch of salt
1 teaspoon extra-virgin olive oil
1–2 tablespoons water

Additional toppings
sliced red onions, soaked in
  gherkin juice for 10 minutes
parsley
lettuce
gherkins, sliced
hot sauce
mayonnaise (see page 65)
mustard

**PER SERVING OF 2 SMASH BURGERS WITH
CHEESE, BACON, TOMATO SAUCE:**
NET CARBS 5g | FIBRE 0g | PROTEIN 34g
FAT 37g | 464kcal

**PER SERVING OF 2 SMASH BURGERS WITH
CHEESE, BACON, TOMATO SAUCE AND
SLIDER:** NET CARBS 8g | FIBRE 3g
PROTEIN 40g | FAT 49g | 623kcal

Smash burgers are typical of American diners and are often served as two patties per bun. Frozen mince is not only less expensive than fresh mince, but it often contains a higher fat percentage, which keeps the meat juicy in a smash burger like this. Otherwise, ask your butcher to coarsely grind chuck meat with a good percentage of fat. Instead of sugary ketchup, whip up this intense tomato sauce; despite its simplicity, it works brilliantly.

To make the sauce, mix the ingredients together in a small bowl to make a ketchup consistency. Spread this over the bun bases or serve on the side.

Heat a large, heavy-based frying pan (with a lid) over a medium heat. Add the fat and, when hot, add the bacon and fry on both sides until just crispy. Transfer the bacon to a plate, leaving the fat in the pan.

Meanwhile, divide the mince into 4 even-sized mounds on a plate. Place the pan over a high heat and add the remaining teaspoon of fat if the pan looks dry. When the fat is shimmering hot, put a mound of mince into the pan. Press it down firmly with a fish slice until it is around 1cm (½ inch) thick and around 8cm (3¾ inchces) wide. Repeat with the other mounds of mince, doing this in two batches if necessary. Season them evenly with the salt and pepper.

Cook the burgers for around 2 minutes or until they are browned and crisp on the bottom. Flip the burgers over and evenly distribute the cheese between two of them. Put the lid on to cook for a further 2–3 minutes, or until the cheese has melted. Remove the pan from the heat and transfer the cheeseless burgers first to the bases of the buns followed by the ones with cheese.

Serve straight away with the bacon, onions, parsley, lettuce, gherkins and hot sauce, mayo or mustard. Top them with the lids and eat as they are or with a green salad.

LAMB ON THE GRILL
WITH ANCHOVY DRESSING

Serves 4

500g (1lb 2oz) lamb steaks or
   1 rack of lamb (separated into
    8 cutlets)
1 tablespoon extra-virgin olive oil
salt and pepper

For the dressing
3 large anchovy fillets in oil
1 garlic clove, peeled
10g (¼oz) parsley leaves and some
   stalks
4 tablespoons extra-virgin olive oil

PER SERVING: NET CARBS 0g | FIBRE 0g
PROTEIN 25g | FAT 27g | 346kcal

This is great cooked on a barbecue where the lamb develops a smoky flavour from the fire, but it also works under a hot grill or pan-fried like the chicken in the Cobb Salad (see page 88). On a barbecue, we sometimes add a little rosemary to the fire to release the flavour.
It is great with the Italian Roast Vegetables (see page 167) or any of the greens. I prefer lean lamb steaks, but the rest of the family like the fat. Splash out with a rack of lamb for a special occasion.

Heat a barbecue or grill to high.

If you are using lamb steaks and they are more than 1cm (½ inch) thick, put them on a chopping board and lay a piece of baking paper over the top. Using a meat mallet, a rolling pin or the base of a small saucepan, bash them until they are 1cm (½ inch) thick.

Season the lamb with salt and pepper and rub each one with the oil, ready for the grill. Set aside on a plate.

Put the anchovies, garlic and parsley together on a chopping board and, using a large knife, finely chop them together. Scrape them into a serving bowl and stir in a generous twist of pepper and the olive oil, a little at a time, until you have a thick sauce. Set aside.

Place the lamb steaks on the barbecue, or place in a tray and cook under the grill, for a couple of minutes on each side until they have browned. Transfer to a warm serving dish and serve the dressing on the side.

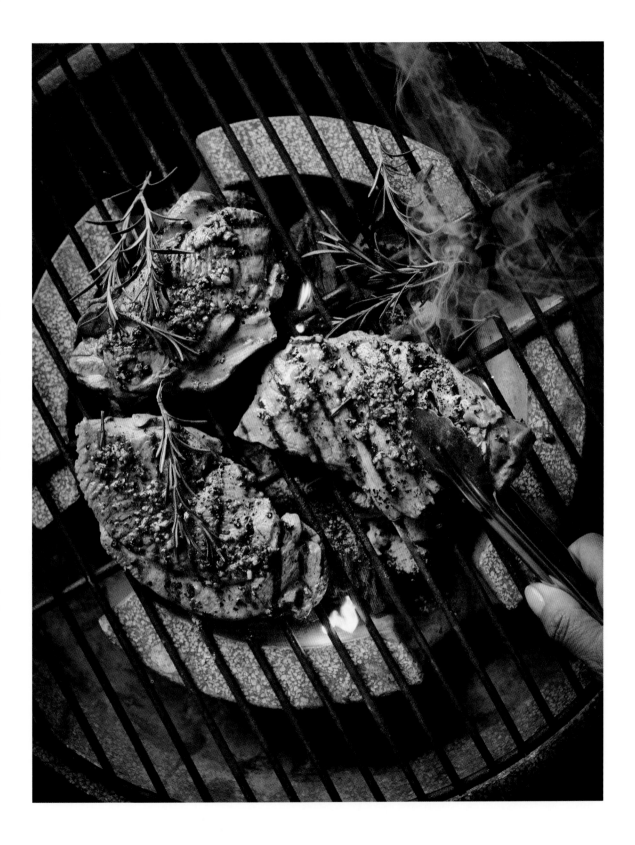

STEAK

Serves 2

2 sirloin steaks, fat trim intact,
(approx. 440g/15½oz total
weight)
1 garlic clove, lightly crushed
few sage leaves
1 sprig of rosemary
salt and pepper
Herb butter (see page 66)

PER SERVING WITH NO BUTTER:
NET CARBS 0g | FIBRE 0g
PROTEIN 66g | FAT 10g | 352kcal

Grass-fed beef from a small farm will be better for you and the environment; however, do try the less expensive cuts such as flat iron or bavette if your butcher will prepare them for you. It is always a good idea to warm them up to room temperature before you start to cook. This ensures a warm centre, even if you like them rare. Allow 20 minutes for this, patting dry with kitchen paper.

I like to use the fat from the edge of the steak, but if you don't have the fatty edge, heat a little ghee or dripping in the pan to cook the steaks.

Season the steaks with salt and pepper. Heat a non-stick frying pan over a high heat.

Hold the 2 steaks together with tongs, with the fat side down, and place in the hot frying pan. Let the fat sizzle, brown and melt; you will soon have a pool of it large enough to cook the steaks.

Now lay the steaks down separately and cook them to your liking (see below). Add the garlic and herbs to the pan while the steaks are cooking. Remove the steaks from the pan and set aside in a warm place to rest for around 10 minutes before serving. In the photo we have served the steak with Herb Butter made with Tarragon (see page 66) and Crunchy Aubergine Chips (see page 157).

How to tell when a steak is done

To give you a guide on timing: a sirloin or rib-eye steak that is 2cm (¾ inch) thick will take about 1½ minutes a side for rare, 2 minutes a side for medium–rare and 3 minutes a side for medium. Or use a meat thermometer poked into the thickest part and measure 45°C (113°F) for rare, 55°C (131°F) for medium–rare, 60°C (140°F) for medium, 65°C (149°F) for medium–well done.

Most chefs use their fingers to tell when a steak is done to their liking, by pressing the top of it while it is still in the pan. The feel shows them how it is

cooked. You can compare the feeling to various parts of your hand, using this guide:

Press the thumb and index finger of one hand together and, with the index finger of the other hand, prod the soft fleshy area at the base of your thumb. Rare steak will be soft to the touch like this. Press your middle finger and thumb together and feel the same point at the base of your thumb. Medium–rare steak will feel like this. Doing the same with the third finger will feel like medium and with the little finger, like well done.

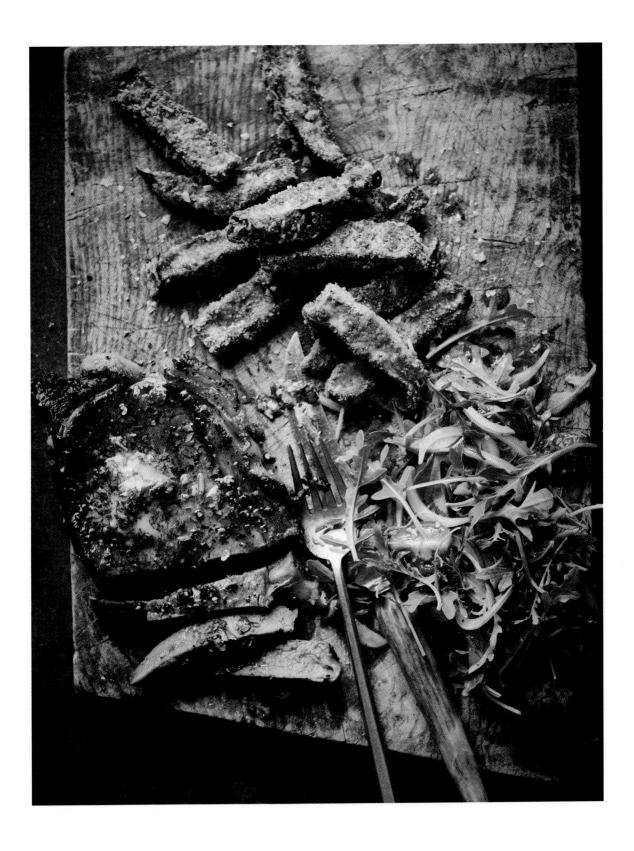

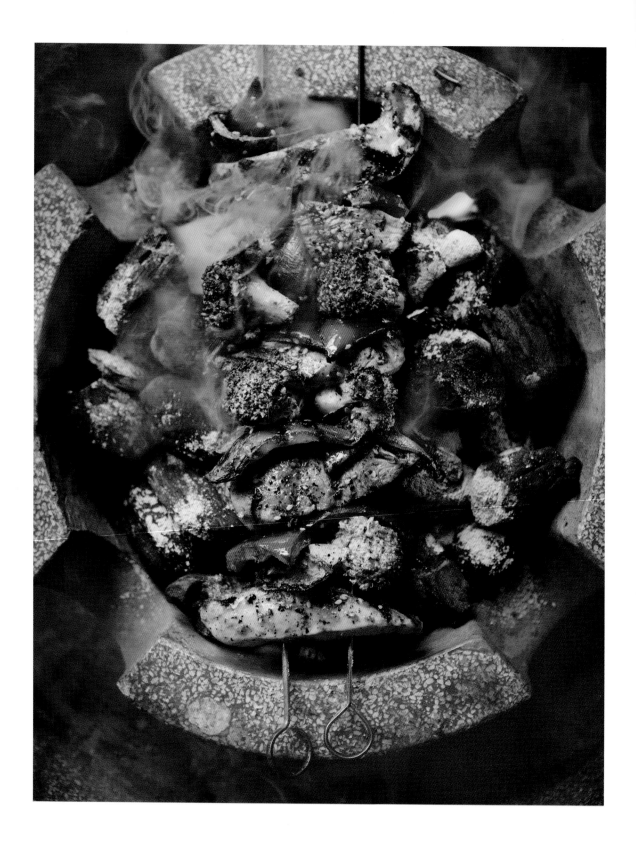

ZA'ATAR CHICKEN

Serves 4

For the marinade
100g (3½oz) 10% fat Greek yoghurt
1 tablespoon extra-virgin olive oil
1 garlic clove, grated
1 tablespoon za'atar mix (see right)
½ teaspoon chilli powder or chilli
    flakes
½ teaspoon salt
plenty of freshly ground black

For the chicken
500g (1lb 2oz) chicken fillets or
    breast, cut into finger-width
    slices
300g (10½oz) broccoli, cut into
    florets
1 onion, cut into wedges
8 cherry tomatoes, halved, or 1 red
    pepper, cored, deseeded and
    cut into 8 strips
3 tablespoons extra-virgin olive oil

To serve
lemon wedges
handful of coriander or parsley,
    roughly chopped

PER SERVING: NET CARBS 11g | FIBRE 5g
PROTEIN 44g | FAT 22g | 437kcal

Za'atar is the Arabic word for a herb from the mint family that is similar to oregano; however, in more recent years, za'atar has come to mean a Levantine spice mix. It is available in most supermarkets, but I prefer to make my own; it takes just minutes and keeps for weeks. You'll find the recipe on our website www.thegoodkitchentable.com. Marinating makes meat more tender, and though doing it the day before helps you get ahead and doesn't harm the dish, you need only 30 minutes to make a difference. The 'longer the better' is a myth, as the marinade can soak only a little way into the meat, however long you leave it.

This easy recipe is great when freshly made, but also makes for good leftovers to pack up and take to work. To make this into a feast, serve the chicken on top of a large platter of green salad, on top of the Hummus on page 70, or with the Homage to Delia Layered Salad on page 164.

Mix the ingredients for the marinade in a large mixing bowl. Add the chicken and broccoli to the bowl and add the onion wedges, using your fingers to break up them up into separate petals. Use a large spoon to stir everything through. Cover and leave in the refrigerator for 30 minutes or up to overnight.

Heat the grill to hot – around 230°C (450°F) is ideal. Line a baking sheet with foil or a silicone baking mat. Alternatively, light your barbecue.

If using a grill, lay the chicken mixture, cherry tomatoes or peppers in a single layer on the lined baking sheet. Drizzle over the oil.

If using a barbecue, thread the marinated ingredients and the peppers onto two skewers and drizzle with oil.

Grill the chicken and vegetables for 12–15 minutes or until it is charred at the edges. Turn the pieces, move the onions around and grill for a further 5 minutes, or until the chicken is cooked through and no longer pink inside when you cut into the thickest piece. If you have a thermometer, it should measure 75°C (167°F).

Serve the chicken hot or at room temperature with the herbs and lemon wedges.

PASTA ALTERNATIVES

On these pages are our imaginative ways to swap pasta for non-starchy vegetables to drastically cut the carbs. Also check out the Leek paccheri on page 10. They saved Giancarlo from his lack of pasta when he first went low carb. He could eat all the traditional sauces and not raise his blood glucose levels. If you are higher on the CarbScale (see page 38) and are finding it hard to give up pasta, try adding a small portion of pasta to your veggie alternatives. For our sons, I like to cook 25g (1oz) dried weight of spelt pasta per person and add this to the veggies; it gives bite and texture to the plate.

SWOODLES WITH SAGE BUTTER

Serves 2

400g (14oz) swede
1 tablespoon ghee or butter
1 garlic clove, lightly crushed
a few sage leaves
100ml (3½fl oz) water
salt and pepper

PER SERVING: NET CARBS 13g
FIBRE 5g | PROTEIN 2g
FAT 6g | 124kcal

Buttery spirals of swede are packed with flavour as they are fried with sage and garlic. Perfect for enjoying with any pasta sauce, with fried eggs or as a side to sausages. Compared to a similar serving of wheat spaghetti, which contains 30g (1oz) of net carbs, swoodles have far fewer carbs and 3 times the fibre, making them a brilliant swap.

Peel the swede and cut into pieces around 5 × 5 × 12cm (2 × 2 × 4½ inches) so it will fit into the spiralizer (the peelings can be kept or frozen for a stock). Fit each swede piece on a spiralizer with a medium cutter and push it through to form strands like thick spaghetti. Cut them into manageable lengths with a pair of scissors.

Heat the ghee or butter in a large frying pan (with a lid) over a medium–high heat. Add the garlic and sage and fry until you can smell them. Add the swoodles, some salt, plenty of pepper and the measured water, and put the lid on. Cook for 8–10 minutes until they have softened, shaking the pan from time to time and giving them a stir a couple of times.

Serves 2

350g (12oz) Lamb Ragu (see page 124)
2 tablespoons double cream
   (optional)
1 quantity Swoodles with Sage
   Butter, hot
25g (1oz) Pecorino or Parmesan
   cheese, finely grated, to serve

PER SERVING INCLUDING CREAM AND CHEESE: NET CARBS 17g | FIBRE 7g
PROTEIN 41g | FAT 43g | 644kcal

Swoodles with Lamb Ragu
Heat the lamb ragu in a small saucepan with the cream, if using. Pour over the hot swoodles and serve with the Pecorino on top. See photo on cover.

BUTTERED CABBAGE RIBBONS

This is a really good alternative to ribbons of pasta such as pappardelle or fettuccine (they even look like them), so they are perfect with meaty sauces like ragu. Any cabbage can be transformed into soft, tender ribbons; white cabbage is firmer and will take a couple of minutes longer than cavolo nero, while young green leaves of pointed or Savoy cabbage take just 2–3 minutes.

Serves 2

400g (14oz) white, sweetheart or Savoy cabbage
1 tablespoon salted butter
4 tablespoons water
salt and pepper

PER SERVING:
NET CARBS 7g | FIBRE 5g | PROTEIN 3g | FAT 5g | 101kcal

Discard any outer bruised leaves of the cabbage, then cut it in half and chop away the tough core. Lay the cabbage flat-side down on a chopping board and use a sharp knife to cut slices around 1cm (½ inch) wide. Pull the slices apart to form ribbons.

To cook the cabbage ribbons, put them into a medium saucepan with the butter, measured water and some seasoning and cover with a lid. Cook over a medium heat for 5–10 minutes or until tender and translucent, adding a splash more water if they look dry. Drain before serving with the sauce of your choice.

COURGETTI

Courgetti, strands of spiralized courgette, has been popular for some years now. It is light on carbs and calories and its delicate flavour is perfect with almost any pasta sauce. The strands can be stirred into a hot sauce to wilt them or cooked as in the recipe below. Enjoy them in place of linguine or spaghetti. These are also ideal with ragu.

Serves 2

1–2 courgettes (approx. 300g/10½oz total weight)
2 tablespoons extra-virgin olive oil
1 garlic clove, peeled and lightly squashed
few slices of hot red chilli or pinch of chilli flakes
   (optional)

PER SERVING:
NET CARBS 4g | FIBRE 2g | PROTEIN 3g | FAT 14g | 153kcal

Put the courgettes through a spiralizer on the finer cutter setting to form long strands, like tagliolini. With a pair of scissors, give them a haircut to shorten them to about the length of a cook's knife. This is so you can easily twiddle them around a fork when eating.

To cook the courgetti, heat the extra-virgin olive oil with the garlic clove and chilli, if using, in a large frying pan or saucepan over a gentle heat. Add the courgetti and pan-fry, tossing the strands in the oil with tongs for just 2 minutes to warm them up. Use tongs to remove them from the pan, leaving any liquid from the courgetti and the garlic in the pan, and stir into a warm sauce of your choice.

SAUSAGE AND MUSHROOM TRAYBAKE PASTA SAUCE

Serves 4

6 high-meat-content sausages
400g (14oz) chestnut or wild mushrooms, trimmed and thickly sliced
2 garlic cloves, unpeeled and lightly crushed
100ml (3½fl oz) dry white wine or water
4 tablespoons extra-virgin olive oil
handful of sprigs of thyme pinch of salt
pinch of freshly ground black pepper
35g (1¼oz) Parmesan or other hard cheese
125g (4½oz) crème fraîche or soured cream
1 quantity Buttered Cabbage Ribbons (see page 106) or other pasta alternative

PER SERVING: NET CARBS 4g | FIBRE 1g PROTEIN 23g | FAT 42g | 506kcal

PER SERVING WITH BUTTERED CABBAGE RIBBONS: NET CARBS 12g | FIBRE 6g PROTEIN 26g | FAT 48g | 606kcal

To keep the carbs down look for high-meat-content sausages, such as Heck sold in the UK, rather than those filled with rusk or flour. This creamy sausage pasta sauce is a hit served on traditional pasta mixed with vegetables or just Buttered Cabbage Ribbons or Swoodles (see pages 106 and 107).

Heat the oven to 240°C/220°C fan (475°F), Gas Mark 9.

Peel the skin away from the sausages and break them into bite-sized pieces in a large mixing bowl. Add the mushrooms, garlic, wine, oil, half the thyme and the seasoning and mix together so that all the ingredients are coated.

Spread out the mixture in a single layer on a large baking tray and put in the oven to roast for 18–20 minutes, or until the sausages are lightly browned.

Meanwhile, shave the Parmesan with a vegetable peeler. When the sausages are ready, remove the tray from the oven and randomly dot spoonfuls of the crème fraîche over the tray. Scatter over the Parmesan shavings and remaining thyme sprigs. Put the tray back into the oven and cook for 3 minutes, or until the cheese has melted.

Cook your Buttered Cabbage Ribbons or other pasta alternative and put in warm serving bowls. Pour the sauce on top. Serve straight away.

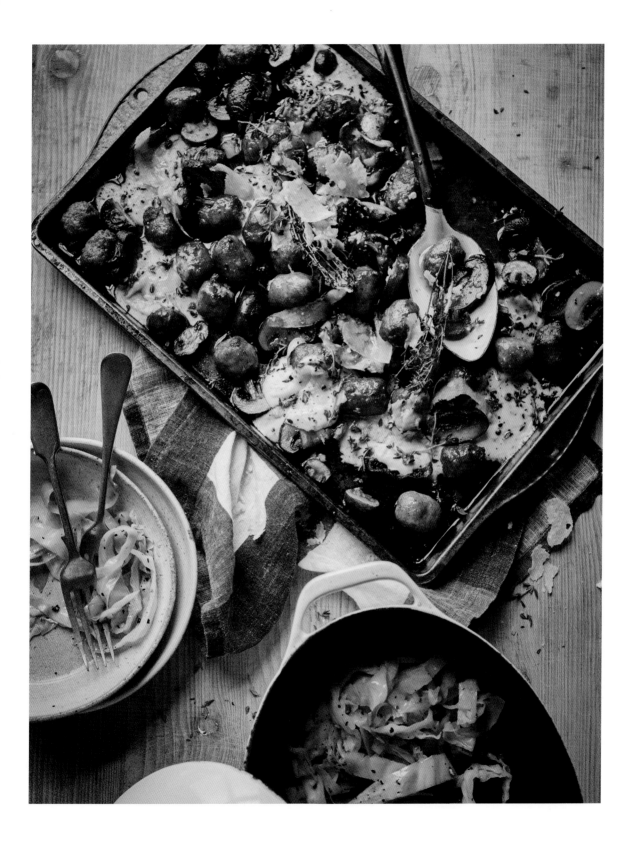

LEEK PACCHERI WITH CHEESY BEAN OR CHICKEN SAUCE

Serves 2

For the leek paccheri
500g (1lb 2oz) leeks, trimmed, cleaned and cut into 2cm- (¾-inch-) thick rounds
4 tablespoons warm water
10g (¼oz) butter
salt and pepper

For the sauce
½ quantity of either the Classic Italian or the Quick Tomato Sauce (see page 64)
3 tablespoons double cream
235g (8¼oz) butter beans, drained, or cooked chicken, chopped
25g (1oz) Parmesan cheese, finely grated
basil leaves, to serve

PER SERVING OF LEEK PACCHERI:
NET CARBS 13g | FIBRE 2g | PROTEIN 2g
FAT 4g | 95kcal

PER SERVING OF CHEESY BEAN SAUCE: NET CARBS 20g | FIBRE 10g
PROTEIN 10g | FAT 26g | 374kcal

PER SERVING OF CHEESY CHICKEN SAUCE: NET CARBS 9g | FIBRE 4g
PROTEIN 29g | FAT 29g | 413kcal

The pasta paccheri, pronounced 'pakkery', derives its name from the word 'slaps' in Italian, believed to be due to the sound it makes when eaten or tossed in sauce. In this case, the pasta is replaced by tubes of leek, which are not only low in carbs, but add a wonderful flavour to any dish. I give the option of adding beans or chicken for protein – any other beans or chickpeas are also good with this, as is any leftover meat.

With your finger, push the centre of the cut leeks to separate the rings. Drop them into a medium saucepan as you do this. Don't worry if a few stay together. Add the warm water, butter and seasoning, and cover with a lid. Bring to the boil, then reduce the heat to simmer for 7 minutes, or until the leeks are tender but still green. Shake the pan frequently during cooking and if they look dry, add a dash more water.

Meanwhile, reheat the tomato sauce in a frying pan over a medium heat. Add the cream, beans or meat and the cheese and stir through until melted.

When the leeks are done, remove the lid and drain through a colander. Use tongs to divide the the leek paccheri between two warm bowls and top with the pasta sauce. Finish with a few basil leaves and serve straight away.

JEN'S TUNA CASSEROLE

Serves 4

3 tablespoons extra-virgin olive oil

1 small onion, finely chopped

400g (14oz) broccoli or
   cauliflower, riced (see page 156)

100ml (3½fl oz) water

400g (14oz) can chopped
   tomatoes

150g (5½oz) tuna in olive oil

100g (3½oz) mature Cheddar
   cheese, coarsely grated

125g (4½oz) mozzarella cheese,
   coarsely grated

1 teaspoon English or Dijon
   mustard

100ml (3½fl oz) double cream

salt and pepper

PER SERVING: NET CARBS 9g | FIBRE 3g
PROTEIN 26g | FAT 36g | 468kcal

This is Jen Unwin's childhood comfort food, which her mum made her. Originally it was made with white rice but now Jen makes it for her grandchildren with broccoli or cauliflower rice and they love it. It makes a great light lunch that the whole family enjoys. The combination of a hot, cheesy topping, tuna and tomatoes is delicious.

Heat the oil in a medium frying pan (with a lid) over a gentle heat. Add the onion and fry for 7–10 minutes until soft. Add the broccoli rice or cauli-rice and the measured water, then season. Put the lid on the frying pan and cook over a medium heat for around 8 minutes or until the broccoli or cauliflower is soft, checking it a couple of times; you may need a splash more water if things look dry.

Remove the pan from the heat and tip the broccoli or cauliflower into a small flameproof dish. Drain the tomatoes in a sieve to get rid of most of the juice. Season with salt and pepper, then pour over the broccoli rice or cauli-rice. Drain the tuna and flake the fish over the tomatoes.

Heat the oven to 240°C/220°C fan (475°F), Gas Mark 9.

Mix the cheeses, mustard, and cream together in a microwave-proof bowl and put into the microwave on full power for 1 minute. Stir until smooth or microwave for another 30 seconds. If you don't have a microwave, heat the sauce in a small pan over a medium heat and stir until melted. Pour the cheese sauce over the tuna mixture.

Bake for around 20 minutes or until browned and bubbling. Remove from the oven and serve straight away with a green salad or green vegetables.

LOW-CARB SWAP

SHOP-BOUGHT LASAGNE

(250G/8¾OZ)

54G CARBS

VS

LASAGNE (PAGE 120)

(250G/8¾OZ)

12G CARBS

The joy of batch cooking is that there is always something delicious, low carb and inexpensive waiting in the fridge or the freezer when we're short of time. This way I am never tempted to order a food delivery. I love an organized and full freezer! I've currently got frozen portions of Chicken Curry, Beef Stew, Spinach Sheets for Wraps and Lasagne – they're ready meals, but they are my healthy ready meals. I also slice and freeze my low-carb bread, taking out a slice at a time to use.

The recipes in this chapter serve eight, but I'll often make double the recipe and then freeze the remainder in one or two person portions.

To avoid too much plastic I wrap foods in baking paper fastened with elastic bands, or glass containers with plastic lids. Always allow a bit of extra room in the container as liquids expand when frozen. Double wrapping foods tightly will stop ice forming and freezer burn. If I use plastic bags, I wash them out thoroughly and reuse them. Label everything – you think you will remember but you rarely do!

BATCH & FREEZE

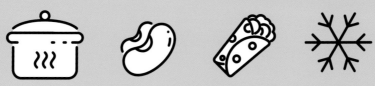

SIMPLE BEEF STEW

Serves 12
(makes approx. 3kg/6lb 8oz)

25g (1oz) butter
3 tablespoons extra-virgin olive oil
1 red onion, roughly chopped
3 celery sticks, roughly chopped
2 large carrots, roughly chopped
1.5kg (3lb 5oz) stewing beef
7 sage leaves (approx. 5g/⅛oz)
10g (¼oz) rosemary needles, stems
    discarded
1–2 teaspoons salt and plenty of
    pepper
300ml (10fl oz) red wine
2 tablespoons tomato purée
2 × 400g (14oz) cans Italian plum
    tomatoes

PER SERVING: NET CARBS 4g | FIBRE 2g
PROTEIN 34g | FAT 24g | 399kcal

Buy the best-quality beef you can, preferably grass-fed, also known as pasture-fed, as this ensures the cattle were outdoors at least part of the year; however, this stew is ideal for using economical cuts such as chuck or skirt. This recipe is based on one shown to me by our Tuscan friend Lorenzo Biagi who was just 16 at the time. He serves it with a delicious, zingy gremolata on top.

Although the base flavours are Mediterranean, it is ideal to turn into a Chilli Con Carne or Beef Curry at a later date, as the stew is large enough to divide into six portions of approximately 500g (1lb 2oz); each will feed two. Add lentils or beans to make the stew go further, but note the adjustment in carbs if you do. Other less carby options you could add are mushrooms or swede.

Heat the butter and oil in a heavy-based casserole over a medium heat. Add the onion, celery and carrots and fry for 10 minutes, or until soft.

Add the meat and brown all over for around 20 minutes over a high heat, or until the liquid from the meat has evaporated.

Now make a little pile of the sage leaves, rosemary, salt and pepper and use a large knife to chop them together. This is called a battuto and it should be a finely chopped mixture. Add this to the pan and stir through before pouring in the wine. Let it bubble for a few minutes to lose the strong taste of alcohol. Add the tomato purée and stir through. Next add the tomatoes and then bring to the boil. Bash the tomatoes up with a wooden spoon.

Turn the heat down to a simmer, put a lid on, ajar, and cook for 1¾–2 hours, or until the sauce has reduced and the meat is very tender. Add a little hot water if looks dry at any stage. If the stew is very watery, remove the lid completely and let the water evaporate as it bubbles.

Serve the stew topped with Gremolata, or transform into Curry, Chilli Con Carne or Curry (pages 116–117). All pictured opposite.

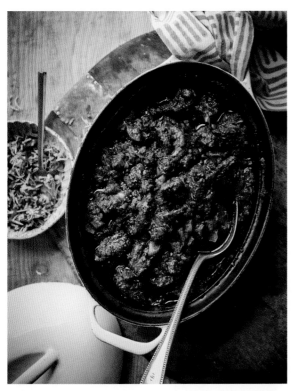
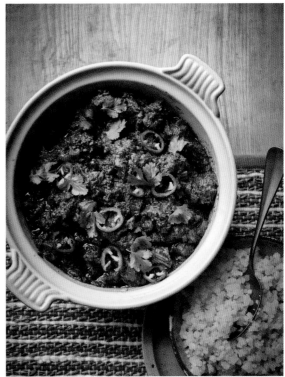
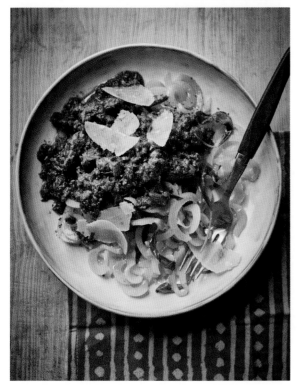
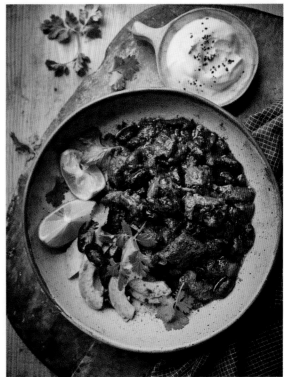

BEEF STEW WITH GREMOLATA

Gremolata is a finely chopped mixture of citrus and soft herbs that gives a wonderful pop of flavour to whatever it lands on. Italians use it on rich stews such as this stew and *Osso Buco*, to cut through heavy sauces. Pictured above left on page 115.

Serves 2

5 teaspoons chopped flat-leaf parsley
1 teaspoon finely pared lemon zest
1 garlic clove, finely chopped
approx. 500g (1lb 2oz) Simple Beef Stew (see page 114)

PER SERVING: NET CARBS 6g | FIBRE 2g
PROTEIN 38g | FAT 33g | 500kcal

To make the gremolata, mix the parsley, lemon zest and garlic in a bowl.

Reheat the beef stew until it is bubbling, then serve out and top with the gremolata.

BEEF CURRY

When the prep and planning is done, you can whip up a homemade curry in no time after work. I love to defrost a portion of the beef stew and turn it into this deliciously warming beef curry with my favourite curry paste. Serve it with cauliflower rice and fresh coriander, the Raita on page 71 and people will think you have slaved away for hours. I like Patak's Madras curry base, but do look for flavours you like; read the ingredients and add according to the ratios they suggest. Sometimes you need only a few tablespoons and others you need to use half a jar of paste to get the flavour correct. Bulk out the curry with non-starchy vegetables such as broccoli or cauliflower florets, or if you are higher on the CarbScale (see page 38), add a tin of lentils or butter beans. Pictured above right on page 115.

Serves 2

approx. 500g (1lb 2oz) Simple Beef Stew (see page 114)
400g (14oz) full-fat coconut milk
curry paste or powder, to taste

Optional additions
Cauli-rice (see page 156)
coriander, roughly chopped
green chilli, sliced (optional)
Cucumber Raita (see page 71)

PER SERVING: NET CARBS 16g | FIBRE 6g
PROTEIN 40g | FAT 25g | 492kcal

Reheat the beef stew with the coconut milk and curry paste until it is bubbling.

Reduce the heat and cook for around 20 minutes until the sauce is thick. Taste and adjust the seasoning to your liking. Enjoy it with Cauli-rice, a sprinkling of coriander, chilli (if using) and a dollop of Raita.

BEEF RAGU ON SWOODLES

A meat sauce, known as a ragu in Italian, doesn't have to be made from minced meat like a Bolognese. Many ragus are made with a whole piece of beef or larger pieces like this recipe. Giancarlo adds cream to the beef stew to thin it down into a rich, sticky ragu and loves it over the Swoodles with Sage Butter (see page 106) or Courgetti with Parmesan (see page 107). Pictured below left on page 115.

Serves 2

approx. 500g (1lb 2oz) Simple Beef Stew (see page 114)
2 tablespoons double cream (optional)
1 quantity Swoodles with Sage Butter (see page 106), hot
25g (1oz) Parmesan or Grana Padano cheese, finely grated or shaved
salt and pepper

PER SERVING: NET CARBS 19g | FIBRE 7g | PROTEIN 40g | FAT 39g | 625kcal

Reheat the beef stew until it is bubbling, adding enough water to give it a sauce consistency and break up any larger pieces of meat with a wooden spoon. You can also take 2 forks to the stew to break up the meat, giving a pulled appearance. Add the cream, if using. Taste and adjust the seasoning to your liking.

Serve over the swoodles, topped with the cheese.

CHILLI CON CARNE

By serving the chilli in bowls with soured cream and grated cheese, you won't notice the missing rice or bread. Adding beans is traditional and bumps up the quantity; however, it doubles the carbs, hence only adding half a can. The other half can be frozen for another day. If it's quantity you are after, add more non-starchy vegetables such as celery, mushrooms or pumpkin when making the beef stew. Pictured below right on page 115.

Serves 2

approx. 500g (1lb 2oz) Simple Beef Stew (see page 114)
¼–½ teaspoon hot chilli powder
½ teaspoon ground cumin
½ teaspoon dried oregano
½ teaspoon cinnamon
125g (4½oz) canned kidney beans or black beans (approx. ½ × 400g/14oz can, drained), optional

To serve

flesh of 1 avocado, sliced or mashed
small handful of coriander leaves and stalks, chopped
1 lime, cut into wedges
soured cream
grated Cheddar or feta cheese
Cauli-rice (see page 156)

PER SERVING:
NET CARBS 4g | FIBRE 2g | PROTEIN 34g | FAT 29g | 399kcal
PER SERVING WITH BEANS:
NET CARBS 16g | FIBRE 6g | PROTEIN 40g | FAT 25g | 492kcal

Reheat the beef stew until it is bubbling.

Add the spices, the beans, if using, and enough water to give it a stew consistency. Reduce the heat and cook for around 20 minutes until the sauce is thick. Taste and adjust the seasoning to your liking. Enjoy on its own in a bowl with avocado, coriander, lime, soured cream and grated cheese, or with additional Cauli-rice.

SPINACH SHEETS

Serves 6

Makes 2 sheets (approx.
   30 × 36cm/12 × 14 inches)
or 24 lasagne sheets (approx.
   9 × 7.5cm/4 × 3 inches)
or 4 tortillas (approx. 18 × 30cm/
   7 × 12 inches)
or 12 wraps (approx. 13 × 15cm/
   5 × 6 inches)

extra-virgin olive oil, for greasing
approx. 350g (12¾oz) defrosted or
   cooked spinach, squeezed dry
   through a thin tea towel (from a
   900g/2lb bag of frozen spinach)
½ teaspoon salt
4 eggs
100ml (3½fl oz) almond or full-fat
   cows' milk
10g (¼oz) psyllium husks (see note
   on page 172)

PER TORTILLA (¼ SHEET): NET CARBS 3g
FIBRE 5g | PROTEIN 11g | FAT 7g |
136kcal

PER WRAP (⅙ SHEET): NET CARBS 1g
FIBRE 2g | PROTEIN 4g | FAT 2g |
46kcal

These are one of my most popular creations – a thin sheet made from spinach and egg that can be used instead of pasta for lasagne, cannelloni, burritos, wraps or even spiralled around a filling for pinwheel sandwiches.

We usually use bags of frozen leaf spinach for this. They are sold in 900g–1kg (2–2lb 4oz) bags and, to give you a guide, 900g (2lb) of frozen spinach becomes approximately 350g (12¾oz) once it is defrosted and thoroughly squeezed. Look for frozen leaf spinach as chopped spinach is harder to squeeze.

Line 2 large oven trays or baking sheets measuring around 30 × 40cm (12 x 16 inches) with baking paper and grease each one well with olive oil. Don't worry if you don't have large trays; just prepare more than 2. Prepare another piece of oiled baking paper the same size as your trays; this will be your top sheet.

Whizz all the ingredients together in a food processor until the spinach is finely chopped and you have formed a paste. Divide the mixture between the lined trays. Put the extra sheet of baking paper over the spinach on one tray and carefully press it out to form a thin rectangle measuring roughly 27 × 34cm (10¾ × 13¼ inches) and about 5mm (¼ inch) thick. Carefully peel off the top piece of baking paper. Straighten the spinach along the edges and even it out as necessary with a flat-ended tool such as a fish slice or dough scraper.

Heat the oven to 220°C/200°C fan (425°F), Gas Mark 7.

Repeat making the second spinach sheet with the other tray, reusing the top sheet.

Bake for 8–10 minutes or until the spinach sheets are firm to the touch and set through. Remove from the oven and leave to cool on the tray. Peel the spinach sheets off the paper and cut them to size, depending on how you plan to use them.

The pasta sheets can be kept rolled in the baking paper they were cooked on, covered and either refrigerated for up to 3 days or frozen for 3 months. Defrost overnight in the refrigerator or for an hour at room temperature.

Use your Spinach Sheets to make Spinach Wraps (page 120), Lasagne (page 121) or Spicy Beef Burritos (page 122). All pictured opposite.

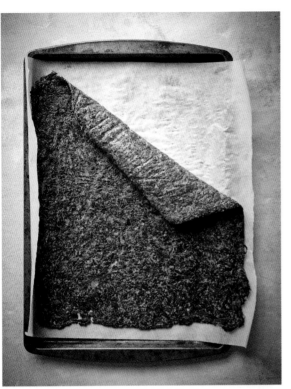
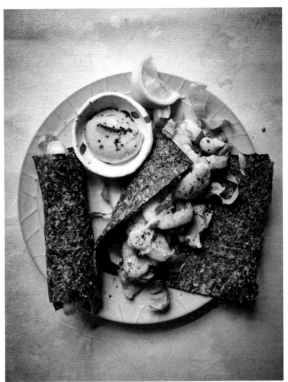
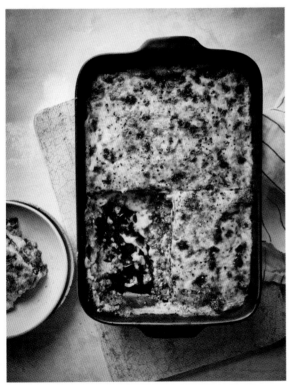
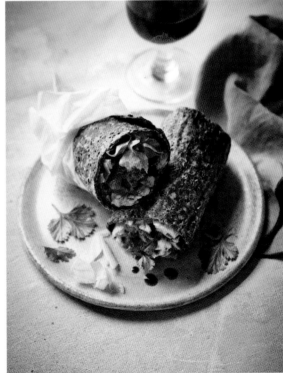

SPINACH WRAPS

Now you can make a homemade alternative to ultra-processed wraps by using 1 Spinach Sheet (see page 118) cut into 6 pieces to make the wraps. This is a great way to use up leftover sauces and ingredients from the refrigerator. The wraps can be wrapped in baking paper and taken to work, on picnics or to school. Pictured above right on page 119.

A few hints and filling suggestions:

- Eat the wraps cold or warm them in the microwave on full power for 10 seconds, or dry-fry them in a pan for the same time. Fillings are good warm or cold.

- It's a good idea to include a sauce to help stick the wrap together.

- Allow 2 wraps per person or add a healthy dessert to make these a lunch or dinner.

- Think about varying the texture with crunchy lettuce, chopped nuts, soft avocado or grated carrot and something to bite into like chicken, bacon or shredded meats.

- To give flavour, season the filling and add a squeeze of lemon or a dash of hot sauce before wrapping.

- If it looks dry before you wrap, add a teaspoon of extra-virgin olive oil.

- If you aren't eating the wraps straight away, they will keep in the refrigerator for up to a day.

To make a wrap, spread the filling from one edge of the wrap toward the other allowing a border of 1cm (½ inch) on each side. Use any sauce or a little mayo to help the wrap stay closed.

Serve straight away or wrap and chill for up to a day.

SEAFOOD WRAP

1 Spinach Wrap (see left)
¼ avocado, sliced
30g (1oz) Avo Non-mayo (see page 72) or Marie-Rose Sauce (see page 151)
50g (1¾oz) cooked peeled prawns or tuna
25g (1oz) shredded lettuce or cress
squeeze of lemon juice

PER WRAP:
NET CARBS 4g | FIBRE 3g | PROTEIN 17g | FAT 10g | 180kcal

CHEESE AND SPICE WRAP

1 Spinach Wrap (see left)
1 heaped tablespoon Romesco (see page 67)
35g (1¼oz) feta cheese, crumbled
25g (1oz) shredded lettuce
¼ teaspoon black onion (nigella) seeds

PER WRAP:
NET CARBS 3g | FIBRE 3g | PROTEIN 10g | FAT 18g | 228kcal

BREAKFAST WRAP

1 Spinach Wrap (see left)
2 bacon rashers
1 fried egg
1 teaspoon Dijon mustard
25g (1oz) baby spinach leaves

PER WRAP:
NET CARBS 2g | FIBRE 2g | PROTEIN 16g | FAT 16g | 228kcal

OTHER FILLINGS

hummus, harissa and grated carrot
egg mayonnaise and cress
warmed roasted vegetables, mozzarella and basil

LASAGNE

Serves 8

1kg (2lb 4oz) Lamb or Beef Ragu
  (see page page 124)
50g (1¾oz) Parmesan cheese,
  finely grated
1 Spinach Sheet (see page 118)

**For the béchamel (makes approx.
  570g/1lb 4½oz)**
550ml (1 pint) full-fat milk
4 tablespoons cornflour
½ teaspoon salt
¼ teaspoon freshly grated nutmeg
50g (1¾oz) butter, roughly
  chopped
1 bay leaf
freshly ground black pepper

PER SERVING: NET CARBS 12g | FIBRE 3g
PROTEIN 17g | FAT 26g | 363kcal

Giancarlo was devastated to be told he was gluten intolerant as well as diabetic, meaning that pasta was definitely off the menu for good. However, with our Spinach Sheets (see page 118), he can once again indulge in his comfort food, lasagne, baked just as mamma used to make. Pictured below left on page 119.

To make the béchamel, whisk the cornflour into the milk in a cold saucepan with the salt, some pepper and the nutmeg. Add the butter and bay leaf and put the saucepan over a medium-high heat. Cook, while whisking to combine, until it has thickened and is bubbling, about 10 minutes. Season to taste.

Heat the oven to 200°C/180°C fan (400°F), Gas Mark 6..

Drop spoonfuls of one-third of the béchamel and half the ragu on the base of a lasagne dish measuring approximately 22 × 26cm (8½ × 10½ inches). Don't mix them together. Now scatter over a third of the Parmesan. Cut half the spinach sheet into shapes to fit your dish. It could be in one single sheet, rectangles or other shapes, but try to avoid too much overlapping.

Do the same again, finishing with a layer of béchamel and cheese. Bake for 30 minutes. Let the lasagne settle for at least 15 minutes before enjoying it.

SPICY BEEF BURRITOS

Serves 2

½ Spinach Sheet (see page 118),
   approx. 18 × 30cm/7 × 12 inches)
300g (10½oz) Chilli Con Carne
   (see page 117), reheated, or
   other protein-rich filling
20g (¾oz) Cheddar or feta cheese,
   coarsely grated
25g (1oz) shredded lettuce
2 tablespoons Avo Non-mayo (see
   page 72) or soured cream
small handful of coriander or
   parsley, roughly chopped
   (optional)

PER BURRITO: NET CARBS 7g | FIBRE 5g
PROTEIN 28g | FAT 22g | 365kcal

I have recently discovered that half a Spinach Sheet (see page 118) makes an excellent 'tortilla' for a burrito, a food I love but rarely eat due to the flabby, ultra-processed tortillas that upset my stomach! Now I can't stop experimenting with them – try using up leftover Pulled Pork or Fakes base (see pages 146 and 129) or stuffing them with fried eggs, spicy sauce and avocado. They are delicious, portable and filling. They can be as simple or elaborate as you like; try adding fresh herbs, creamy mayo, cheese or salad leaves. Two burritos per person makes a big brunch or one is an ideal light lunch followed by a small dessert. Serve on their own or with salad. Pictured below right on page 119.

Lay a rough rectangle of warm Chilli con Carne into the centre of the tortilla made from half a spinach sheet, leaving a 5cm (2-inch) border around the edge. Top this with the cheese, lettuce, mayo or cream and herbs, if using. Fold in the shorter edges to encase the filling, then tightly roll up the tortilla from one long edge to another. Wrap tightly in a single piece of baking paper to hold it together then cut it in half using a sharp knife. Serve and eat while warm.

SRI LANKAN CURRY PASTE

This is the perfect curry base from my friend Manjula Samarasinghe for beef, chicken, eggs, tofu, fish, chickpeas or prawns which she gave us for our book *The Gentle Art of Preserving*. If you make this and freeze the mixture into 4 portions, you can simply whip up a healthy curry after work in less than 30 minutes.

Makes approx. 460g (1lb)
(enough for 4 curries and each curry serves 4 people)

50g (1¾oz) coriander seeds
5g (⅛oz) cumin seeds
5g (⅛oz) fennel seeds
10–15 fenugreek seeds
1 teaspoon black mustard seeds
1 teaspoon black peppercorns
12 fresh curry leaves
25g (1oz) garlic, finely chopped
25g (1oz) fresh root ginger, finely chopped
2–4 small hot red chillies, finely chopped, to taste
2 onions, roughly chopped
100ml (3½fl oz) cold-pressed rapeseed or extra-virgin olive oil

PER INDIVIDUAL SERVING OF CURRY PASTE:
NET CARBS 2g | FIBRE 2g | PROTEIN 1g | FAT 7g | 78kcal

Put all the spices and the curry leaves in a dry frying pan over a medium heat and toast until they just start to brown and pop, around 5 minutes. Tip on to a plate, or on to a piece of paper folded in half, and leave to cool. Transfer to, or shoot the spice straight from the paper into, a spice grinder or pestle and mortar, and grind them to a powder.

Mix the garlic, ginger, chilli and onion with the oil and then combine with the spices to form a paste. Divide the mixture into 4. Use straight away or freeze in small sealed bags or airtight containers.

CHICKEN CURRY

Manjula uses a jointed chicken but for speed, skinless chicken breasts are perfect. Instead of chicken, add halved hard-boiled eggs, chickpeas or prawns, warm through until piping hot and the prawns are completely pink and cooked through.

Serves 4

1 tablespoon ghee or butter, cold-pressed rapeseed or extra-virgin olive oil
¼ quantity (approx. 115g/4oz) Sri Lankan Curry Paste (see left)
4 skinless chicken breasts, (approx. 830g/1lb 13oz), roughly chopped into bite-sized pieces
400g (14oz) full-fat coconut milk
pinch of chilli flakes (optional)
handful of fresh coriander (optional), to serve
salt and pepper

PER SERVING OF CURRY:
NET CARBS 6g | FIBRE 3g | PROTEIN 39g | FAT 33g | 485kcal

Melt the ghee in a medium saucepan over a medium heat. Add the paste and fry for 5 minutes, stirring constantly. Add the chicken and stir through for 3 minutes until seared all over.

Pour in the coconut milk, rinse out the can with a splash of water and add this, too. Continue to cook, stirring frequently, until the chicken is cooked through; around 15 minutes is usually fine, depending on the size of the pieces. Test a large piece by cutting it in half to make sure it is no longer pink inside.

Taste the curry and adjust the seasoning and chilli heat as necessary. Serve, garnished with coriander if using, alongside Cauli-rice (see page 156) and Cucumber Raita (see page 71).

LAMB RAGU

**Serves 10
(makes approx. 1.75kg/4lb)**

4 tablespoons extra-virgin olive
    oil
1 leek or onion, finely chopped
2 celery sticks, finely chopped
1 red pepper, cored, deseeded
    and finely chopped, or 1 large
    carrot, finely chopped
2 sprigs of rosemary
2 garlic cloves, lightly crushed
2 teaspoons salt
1kg (2lb 4oz) 15–20%-fat minced
    lamb
500g (1lb 2oz) minced pork or
    minced lamb
250ml (9fl oz) dry white wine
2 tablespoons tomato purée
2 × 400g (14oz) cans chopped
    tomatoes
freshly ground black pepper

PER SERVING: NET CARBS 4g | FIBRE 2g
PROTEIN 35g | FAT 25g | 403kcal

Frozen mince is excellent for this; it often has a high fat content, which gives a great flavour. This is perfect as a ragu on courgetti pasta, made into Shepherd's Pie, Moussaka or pilaf with cauliflower rice (see pages 126, 127 and 128). You can also make this recipe with minced beef instead of lamb. I like to add minced pork, as it adds flavour and fat to lamb.

Heat the oil in a large, deep frying pan or saucepan over a medium–low heat. Add the leek or onion, celery, pepper or carrot, rosemary, garlic and seasoning and fry for around 15 minutes, or until softened. Stir and shake the pan frequently; it distributes the vegetables better than simply stirring them.

Add all the meat and brown thoroughly over a high heat while bashing it with a wooden spoon to break up any lumps. Allow any liquid to evaporate and, when the meat is dry, sizzling and starting to stick, it is calling out for the wine, so pour it in.

After 5 minutes, when the wine has reduced, add the tomato purée and canned tomatoes. Rinse the cans out with a little water and add this, too. Bring to the boil, then reduce the heat to a gentle bubble and continue to cook, uncovered for around 1–1½ hours. If the sauce looks a little dry, add a little hot water.

Taste and add more seasoning as necessary, then serve.

Transform your Lamb Ragu into a Shepherd's Pie (page 126), Curried Lamb Pilaf (Page 127) or Moussaka (Page 128). All pictured opposite.

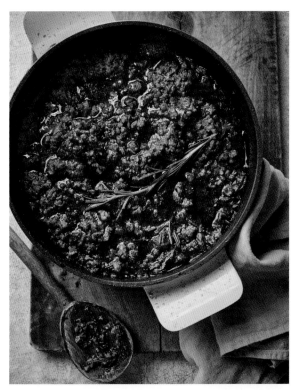
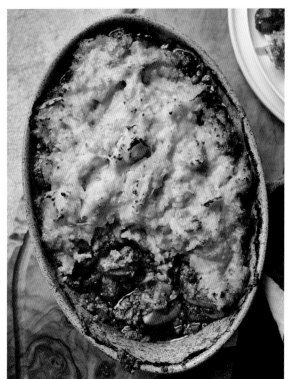
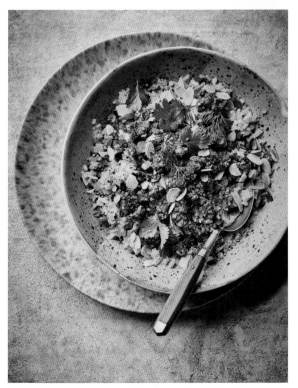
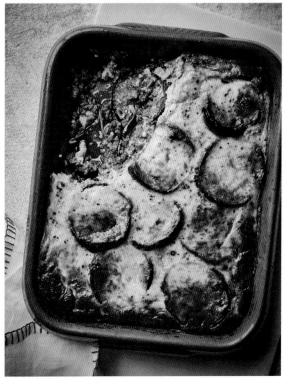

SHEPHERD'S PIE

Serves 4

350g (12oz) celeriac, peeled and
    roughly chopped
40g (1½oz) butter
4 tablespoons double cream
3 tablespoons extra-virgin olive oil
500g (1lb 2oz) chestnut
    mushrooms, trimmed and
    roughly chopped
¼ quantity (approx. 430g/15oz)
    Lamb Ragu (see page 124) or
    Fakes base (see page 129)
1–2 tablespoons Worcestershire
    sauce
50g (2oz) mature Cheddar or
    Parmesan cheese, finely grated
salt and pepper

PER SERVING: NET CARBS 16g | FIBRE 4g
PROTEIN 31g | FAT 44g | 587kcal

Going low carb doesn't mean the end of pies, you will be glad to know. By swapping the potato for celeriac you not only lower the carbs, but increase the flavour of this traditional family favourite. We use one-quarter of the Lamb Ragu recipe, as I like to make the meat go further by adding non-starchy vegetables such as mushrooms. Leftover cooked swede is also good. Alternatively, use half of the Lamb Ragu recipe rather than a quarter. Celeriac is more fibrous than potato, so I find this mash much easier to make with a stick blender. Pictured above right on page 125.

You will need an oven dish measuring approx. 20 × 30cm (8 × 12 inches).

Bring a large pan of salted water to the boil. Add the celeriac and boil for 20–30 minutes until tender. Drain, then add 35g (1¼oz) of the butter along with the cream. Mash with a stick blender or food processor. Taste and season if necessary, then set aside.

Heat the oven to 220°C/200°C fan (425°F), Gas Mark 7.

Heat the oil in a large frying pan and, when hot, fry the mushrooms for 10 minutes or until lightly browned.

Heat the Ragu in a saucepan over a medium heat until piping hot. Add a splash of hot water if it is very thick. Add the Worcestershire sauce to taste, then spoon the meat and mushrooms into the ovenproof dish. Top with dollops of the mash. Use a fork to evenly spread out the mash and create a pattern. Dot the remaining butter and the cheese on top and put into the oven to bake for 25 minutes, or until lightly browned.

Remove from the oven and serve with green vegetables.

CURRIED LAMB PILAF

Serves 4

¼ quantity (approx. 430g/15oz) Lamb Ragu (see page 124) or Fakes base (see opposite)
2–3 teaspoons medium curry powder or curry paste
¼–½ teaspoon chilli flakes
2 teaspoons ground cumin
½ teaspoon ground turmeric
3 tablespoons extra-virgin olive oil
1 onion or leek, finely chopped
500g (1lb 2oz) cauliflower or broccoli, riced (see page 156)
100ml (3½fl oz) hot meat stock, water or leftover gravy, or more if needed
25g (1oz) flaked almonds, toasted
3 tablespoons (approx. 20g/¾oz) roughly chopped herbs (such as coriander, dill or flat-leaf parsley)
salt and pepper

PER SERVING: NET CARBS 9g | FIBRE 5g
PROTEIN 30g | FAT 30g | 424kcal

Grab a container of frozen Lamb Ragu in the morning and let it defrost during the day. In 15 minutes, dinner will be ready, as most of the work will have already been done. While the mince is heating, you can alter the flavour with spices and make the cauliflower rice as an alternative to the traditional white rice. The pilaf is great finished with a lot of herbs; I use a mixture from the refrigerator and what is in the garden, but you could scatter over a couple of teaspoons of dried thyme or oregano if that is all you have. Pictured below left on page 125.

Heat the Lamb Ragu or Fakes base in a saucepan until it is bubbling hot, adding a splash of hot water to loosen it. Add the spices to taste.

To cook the cauli-rice, heat the oil in a large frying pan (with a lid) over a gentle heat. Add the onion or leek and fry for 10 minutes until soft. Add the cauli-rice and the hot meat stock, water or gravy, then season. Put the lid on the frying pan and cook over a medium heat for around 8 minutes, or until the cauliflower is soft, checking it a couple of times; you may need more stock or a splash of water if things look dry. The cauliflower rice should change from bright white grains to soft, cream-coloured ones.

Now add the Ragu to the cauliflower rice and stir through. Taste and add more seasoning, if necessary. Fold in the flaked almonds and herbs and serve straight from the pan into warm bowls.

MOUSSAKA

Serves 4

3 aubergines (approx. 600g/1lb 5oz total weight)
3 tablespoons extra-virgin olive oil
¼ quantity (approx. 430g/15oz) Lamb Ragu (see page 124) or Fakes base (see page 129)
1 teaspoon ground cinnamon
1 teaspoon dried oregano
salt and pepper

For the topping
75g (2½oz) mature Cheddar, Parmesan or Grana Padano cheese, grated
4 large eggs
200ml (7fl oz) 10% fat kefir yoghurt or Greek yoghurt
½ teaspoon freshly grates nutmeg

PER SERVING: NET CARBS 20g | FIBRE 7g
PROTEIN 20g | FAT 22g | 369kcal

PER SERVING WITH FAKES BASE: NET CARBS 22g | FIBRE 8g
PROTEIN 14g | FAT 19g | 330kcal

Defrost 300g (10½oz) Lamb Ragu overnight or during the day and make up a deliciously spicy moussaka in 45 minutes in the evening. Traditional moussaka has layered aubergine and potato separated by a rich lamb sauce. In this version, we have doubled the aubergine instead. If you are keto, omit the aubergines or use only one. For a vegetarian version, use the Fakes base instead of the lamb and stick to Cheddar. Pictured below right on page 125.

Heat the oven to 240°C/220°C fan (475°F), Gas Mark 9.

Cut each aubergine into around 12 circles, just less than 1cm (½ inch) thick, and lay them on a baking tray. Brush with the oil and lightly season with salt and pepper. Bake for 15 minutes, or until the flesh is cooked through and lightly browned. Remove from the oven and set aside.

Meanwhile, mix together the ingredients for the topping in a bowl so that they are well blended. Season with only pepper, as the cheese is salty enough. Set aside.

Heat the Lamb Ragu or Fakes base in a saucepan until it is bubbling hot, adding enough water to make it into a pourable Bolognese-style sauce. Add the cinnamon and oregano. Use a spoon to layer one half of the Ragu into a small ovenproof dish measuring around 20 × 25cm (8 × 10 inches). Lay over half the aubergines, followed by the remaining Ragu and repeat another layer of aubergine.

Pour the topping mixture over the aubergines and bake for 20–25 minutes, or until it has has risen and browned.

FAKES SOUPA

Serves 4 (makes 1kg/2lb 4oz)

For the Fakes base
4 tablespoons extra-virgin olive oil, plus extra to serve
1 carrot, finely diced
1 large celery stick, finely diced
1 small onion, finely diced
2 garlic cloves, roughly chopped
1 bay leaf or sprig of rosemary
250g (9oz) dry, flat green or brown lentils
1 teaspoon ground cumin
1 teaspoon Aleppo chilli flakes or a pinch of regular chilli flakes
150g (5½oz) tomato passata or puréed canned tomatoes
1 tablespoon tomato purée
salt and pepper

For the Fakes Soupa
approx. 600ml (20fl oz) warm vegetable or chicken stock or hot water

Serving suggestions
1 tablespoon red wine vinegar
feta, crumbled, to taste
Kalamata olives, to taste
parsley, chopped, to taste

PER SERVING OF FAKES SOUPA WITHOUT TOPPINGS: NET CARBS 21g | FIBRE 7g PROTEIN 10g | FAT 18g | 293kcal

Pronounced 'fah-kehs', this Greek way to cook flat, greenish-brown lentils makes an earthy, textural backdrop to eggs, fish, pork or chicken. This recipe was shown to me by Anne Hudson, who spends part of her life in Greece and loves this recipe. I can see why, as it is pure comfort food and often eaten during Lent when no meat is consumed. The base can be eaten as a vegan ragu or in a bowl with a couple of fried eggs; as a filling for lasagne, moussaka or a burrito; or with added stock as a soup, as it is here. When served as a 'soupa', if it isn't Lent, it is sometimes finished with feta, parsley and Greek olives. The base makes a perfect vegetarian alternative to the Simple Beef Stew on page 114 the Lamb Ragu on page 124 and can be used as a substitute. Lentils freeze well, so I divide these into four single portions. Some people wash and soak the lentils or boil them separately, but read the instructions on your packet; mine are always fine to cook like this.

Heat the oil in a medium saucepan over a gentle heat. Add the carrot, celery, onion, garlic and bay leaf and cook for 10–15 minutes, until the vegetables are soft. Add the lentils and spices and stir through. Continue to cook for around 7 minutes until they almost catch, to develop the umami flavours. Add the tomato passata, or puréed canned tomatoes, and purée and and stir through – you now have your Fakes base. To turn it into the Soupa add the stock and stir through.

For either the base or Soupa, continue to cook for around 45 minutes–1 hour, or until the lentils are just soft, adding more hot stock or water as necessary if they look dry.

Add seasoning to your taste and serve in warm bowls. At this point it is traditional to add a drizzle of vinegar and olive oil. Other toppings can be added now, such as crumbled feta, olives and parsley.

LOW-CARB SWAP

SHOP-BOUGHT SAGE AND ONION STUFFING

(200G/7OZ)

44G CARBS

VS

SAGE AND ONION STUFFING (PAGE 141)

(200G/7OZ)

6G CARBS

Celebrations are when people often go off the rails. However, with a little forward planning you can still celebrate and feel good afterwards. In this chapter, you will find dishes and drinks that your family and friends will enjoy, without even realizing they are eating low carb. You really can enjoy the party while your body celebrates the lack of glucose spikes!

We have included a Christmas spread with a low-carb bread sauce and stuffing, as well as a couple of cocktail ideas to get the party going.

Most importantly don't give up after any indulgence over festivities, it is bound to happen sometimes. Just get right back on track the next day. Giancarlo and I often put on a couple of kilos on holiday but we lose it within a week of strict low carb once we are back home.

FEASTS & CELEBRATIONS

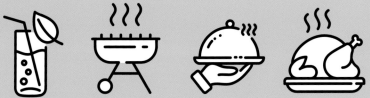

WHAT TO DRINK?

It goes without saying that alcohol has only empty calories and is not nutrient-rich. It can also slow weight loss, as the body tends to burn alcohol before anything else. However, we all like to start the party with a bang, so do try our Raspberry Collins, Remastered or our Smoky Mary (page 147), or look at our suggestions for flavoured water (page 13). A 150ml (5fl oz) glass of brut champagne, very dry cava or very dry Prosecco has around 2g net carbs and a glass of red or dry white is the same. Most importantly don't go for the beer at 13g for a half pint, or the sugary cocktails.

RASPBERRY COLLINS, REMASTERED

Serves 2

40g (1½oz) raspberries
2 sprigs of mint
100ml (3½fl oz) gin
½ teaspoon vanilla extract
juice of ½ lemon
ice
club soda or sparkling water,
    chilled

PER SERVING:
NET CARBS 2g | FIBRE 1g | PROTEIN 0g |
FAT 0g | 129kcal

Between our friend Mike Boynton and our son Giorgio, we had great fun creating cocktails, as you can imagine! The classic Collins cocktail uses sugar syrup to balance a base of gin and lemon juice, but in this version Mike used raspberries and Giorgio added vanilla; between them, they created a refreshing, sparkly blend of sweet fruit and tangy lemon.

In 2 highball glasses, muddle the raspberries and mint together with a cocktail muddler or the handle of a wooden spoon. Add the gin, vanilla and lemon juice, and stir to combine. Add ice to your liking and top up with the club soda. Cheers!

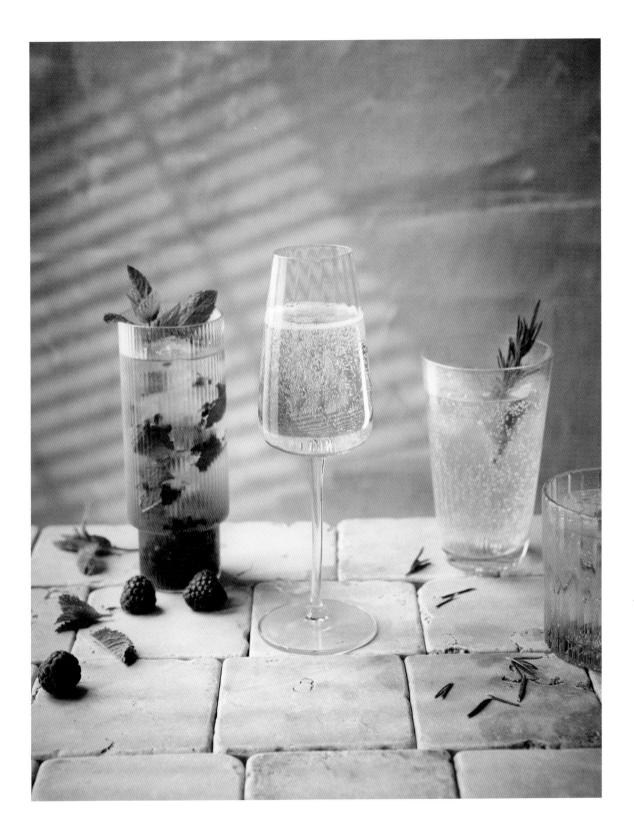

ROMAN CHEESE DIP

Serves 8

100g (3½oz) hazelnuts or pine nuts
2 spring onions or ¼ leek, trimmed, cleaned and roughly chopped
75g (2½oz) herbs (such as coriander, mint, thyme leaves or parsley)
125g (4½oz) feta cheese
5 tablespoons extra-virgin olive oil, plus extra to drizzle
40ml (2½ tablespoons) white or red wine vinegar or cider vinegar, or more to taste
salt and plenty of pepper

PER SERVING: NET CARBS 2g | FIBRE 2g
PROTEIN 4g | FAT 22g | 222kcal

This is based on an ancient Roman recipe written by Columella in the first century CE and translated by Mark Grant in his fascinating book *Roman Cookery*. Columella wrote of 'pounding' the ingredients together like modern-day pesto using 'peppered vinegar', resulting in a textural, creamy paste that is perfect for spreading on the crackers on page 177 or on freshly cut vegetables. As Giancarlo likes to compare himself to a Roman centurion from time to time, I get him to pound this in a pestle and mortar, but you can actually use a food processor for the same result, although don't tell him that! Once this is made, all you need are a few togas and carafes of wine and you are ready to party!

Heat the oven to 220°C/200°C fan (425°F), Gas Mark 7.

Toast the nuts on a tray in the oven for 5 minutes, or until golden brown. Rub any loose skins off the hazelnuts in a folded tea towel. Let them cool before using.

Use your very own Roman centurion or a food processor to pulse together all the ingredients until you have a rough paste. Taste and adjust the flavour with a small pinch of salt, plenty of pepper and vinegar to your liking. Transfer the dip to a shallow bowl, pour over a slick of olive oil and give it a few twists of pepper.

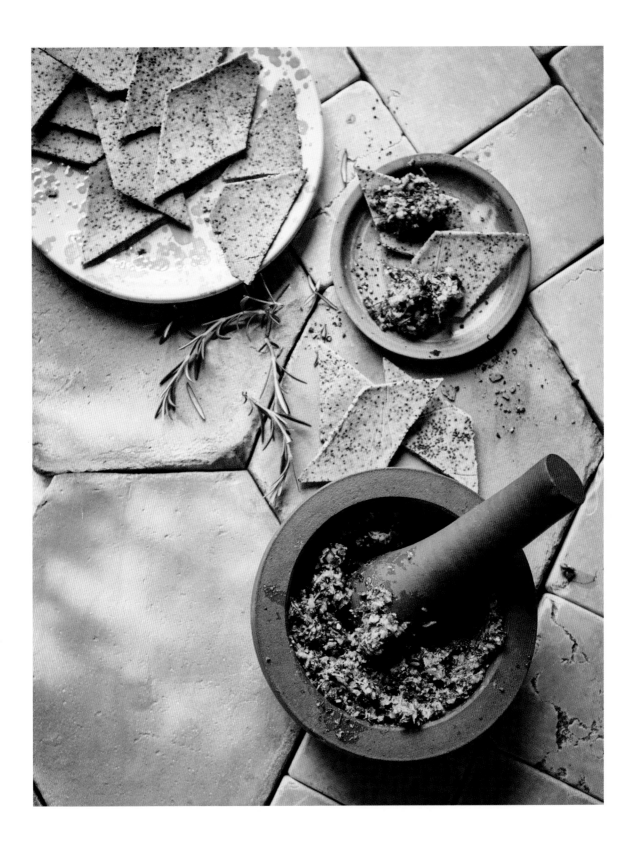

ROAST TURKEY

Serves 12

1 × 6.5kg (14lb 5oz) turkey
1 lemon, halved
few small sprigs of thyme
1 onion, cut into wedges
125g (4½oz) butter, softened
6 smoked streaky bacon rashers
salt and pepper

PER 135G (4¾OZ) SERVING:
NET CARBS 0g | FIBRE 0g | PROTEIN 37g
FAT 22g | 350kcal

I love a traditional Christmas turkey, as after the initial work is done, I can use up the leftovers during the following week by making salads, sandwiches, soups, pies and curries, all with a low-carb twist. Ideally buy a turkey with the giblets, as these will make a wonderful addition in flavour to your gravy. The bird can be prepped a day in advance before cooking. Serve with the Proper Gravy on page 74, the 'Bread' Sauce on page 75, the Roasties on page 166 and the Stir-fried Sprouts with Onion, Bacon and Walnuts on page 160.

Heat the oven to 220°C/200°C fan (425°F) Gas Mark 7. Set a rack in the bottom of the oven, making sure there is space to put the turkey inside.

Lay 2 sheets of foil, one lengthways and the other crossways, on a large roasting tin; make sure they are long enough to go over the top of the turkey and join together, allowing a little space above the breast. Place the turkey on top, crown upward.

Put the lemon, thyme and onion into the cavity, making sure any giblets have been removed. Spread the softened butter over the top of the breast and the thighs, particularly where the skin is thin. Season well all over with salt and pepper.

Bring the foil pieces up and over the turkey, leaving a gap so that the foil only touches the bird around the base and not on top. Fold the foil edges over one another several times to join them together.

Cook the turkey in the oven for 40 minutes. Reduce the oven temperature to 160°C/140°C fan (315°F), Gas Mark 3 and continue to roast for 3½ hours.

Remove the turkey from the oven carefully, so that no juices escape. Increase the oven temperature to 220°C/200°C fan (425°F) Gas Mark 7.

Roll the foil gently down the sides to uncover the turkey; you will reuse this to cover the crown while it is resting later.

Use a large spoon to collect the juices from the tin and pour them over the breast so that they fall down and moisten the bird all over. Lay the streaky bacon slices over the breast. Return the turkey to the hot oven for about 30 minutes until the skin and bacon brown and become crisp.

Use a thermometer to take a reading from the thickest part of the bird to make sure the internal temperature is 75–80°C (167–176°F). Alternatively, pierce the thickest part of the thigh with a sharp knife to make sure the juices run clear; if they are still pink (or the thermometer reads less than 75°C/167°F), then roast for a little longer.

Remove the turkey from the oven and, with help, carefully lift it on to a carving platter. Cover lightly with the foil (removed from the base of the tin) and leave to stand for 30 minutes–1 hour before carving.

Pour the juices from the tin into a jug. When the fat has settled, spoon it off and reserve it for cooking another time. Pure fat will keep at room temperature or in the fridge for weeks. The brown juices below will be packed with flavour and can be added to your gravy or chilled and kept in the refrigerator for up to 3 days to add to a stock. Do taste these juices, however, before using them, as they can be salty.

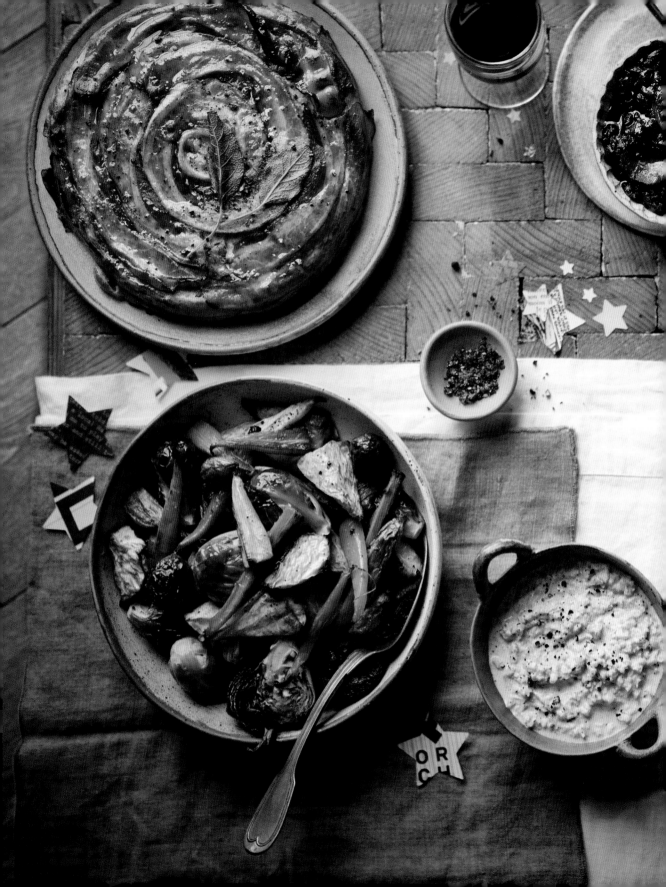

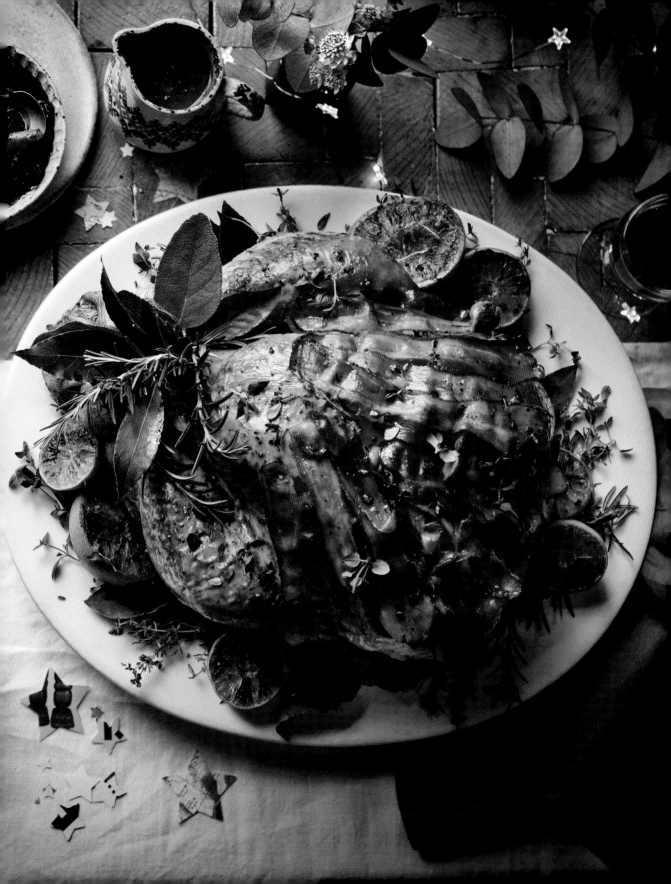

CHICKEN OR TURKEY STOCK

**Makes approx. 2.5 litres
(4½ pints), serves 12**

2kg (4lb 8oz) raw or cooked
    chicken or turkey carcasses or
    bones or fresh chicken wings
1 white onion, cut into eighths
    (don't bother to peel it)
2 large celery sticks, plus any
    leaves, roughly chopped
1 carrot, halved
1 pack giblets (optional)
200ml (7fl oz) white wine
5 litres (9 pints) cold water
1 bay leaf
1 Parmesan cheese rind (optional)

PER SERVING: NET CARBS 1g
FIBRE 2g | PROTEIN 6g
FAT 2g | 50kcal

Making chicken stock for soups or a proper gravy reminds me of my childhood, as my mother would always make it on a Monday after we had roast chicken on Sunday. She and I would pick the meat from the carcass, keeping it to add to other meals. I freeze them until I am making a stock and when I have enough simply add them, frozen, to the pan. As they are cooked, you can skip the roasting stage and boil them with the vegetables. Raw carcasses and bones can be frozen too but should be cooked before making the stock. If you can find giblets, add these; they make a wonderful-tasting stock.

Heat the oven to 220°C/200°C fan (425°F), Gas Mark 7.

Put the raw carcasses, bones or wings into a roasting tin with the vegetables and roast for 1 hour or until well browned but not burnt. If your bones are already cooked, skip this stage.

Remove from the oven and use tongs to transfer the bones and vegetables to a large saucepan with the giblets, if using. Pour any remaining fat from the tin into a bowl for use another time.

Put the roasting tin over a medium heat on the hob and deglaze it with the white wine. Pour this into the saucepan, scraping any brown but not burnt bits in too. Pour over the cold water and bring to the boil. Add the bay leaf and Parmesan rind, if using. Reduce the heat to a very gentle simmer and cook for at least 3 hours and up to 6 hours.

At this point, the stock is ready to use. Simmer for longer if you want a more concentrated stock for freezing. Remove from the heat and strain into a large jug or bowl. Discard everything but the liquid. Use straight away, store in the refrigerator for up to 4 days or freeze for up to 3 months.

SAGE AND ONION STUFFING CAKE

Serves 6

10g (¼oz) butter, for greasing

200g (7oz) thin smoked streaky bacon rashers

1 onion, finely chopped

100g (3½oz) cauliflower, riced (see page 156)

500g (1lb 2oz) minced pork

1 unpeeled apple, cored and finely chopped

2 tablespoons sage leaves, finely chopped, or 1 tablespoon dried sage

2 eggs

½ teaspoon salt

plenty of freshly ground black pepper

PER SERVING: NET CARBS 6g
FIBRE 1g | PROTEIN 24g
FAT 15g | 256kcal

As it is better not to put meat stuffing into the cavity of a bird for fear of it not cooking through, we like to make the stuffing a feature and serve it on the side. For this recipe, it's best to use thin streaky bacon, as it bends easily into a spiral. You can make it without the cauliflower rice, but I found that, like breadcrumbs, the rice softens the pork and adds moisture to stop it from becoming dry. The cake can be prepared in advance and kept in the refrigerator until you are ready to cook it. Any leftovers can be reheated in the oven or microwave. Pictured on page 138.

Butter a 20cm (8-inch) loose-bottomed cake tin. Use the bacon to line the dish in a spiral, laying each rasher flat against the base and starting in the centre. When you reach the edges of the base, push the rashers up slightly to form a corner to seal in the pork. Wind the bacon around the sides, too. If you have any left over, chop it finely and put it into a bowl.

Heat the oven to 200°C/180°C fan (400°F) Gas Mark 6.

Mix the remaining ingredients together thoroughly in the bowl with any leftover bacon. Now pack the mixture into the bacon-lined tin, being careful not to dislodge the rashers.

Bake the stuffing for 30 minutes or until firm to the touch and cooked through. Remove from the oven and cover the tin with a large ovenproof plate or baking tray. Invert the tin so that the stuffing is spiral side up. Wipe away any juices that have leaked out of the meat. Return the cake to the oven for 15–20 minutes to brown.

Serve straight away or keep it warm for up to 30 minutes before serving. Or prepare the cake up to 2 days before serving, then bring it to room temperature for 30 minutes before cooking as above.

LAYERED MUSHROOM, GOATS' CHEESE, PEPPER AND CELERIAC PIE

Serves 8

700g (1lb 9oz) celeriac or swede, peeled and cut into walnut-sized pieces

1½–3 tablespoons ghee or butter

1 onion, finely chopped

2 garlic cloves, finely chopped

1kg (2lb 4oz) wild or chestnut mushrooms, trimmed and roughly sliced

handful of soft sprigs of thyme or 2 teaspoons dried thyme or 3 sprigs of rosemary

200ml (7fl oz) full-fat milk (any kind) or water

250g (9oz) ricotta cheese

350g (12oz) roasted peppers from a jar

200g (7oz) firm goats' cheese or smoked Cheddar cheese

4 sheets of filo pastry

20g (¾oz) melted butter

2 teaspoons sesame seeds

1 teaspoon black onion (nigella) seeds

salt and pepper

PER SERVING: NET CARBS 28g | FIBRE 3g
PROTEIN 16g | FAT 21g | 368kcal

This stunning vegetarian pie is a winner at Christmas or any cold weather feast. There is so much flavour from the gorgeous layers of vegetables. This is one cheat where I allow myself to use ready-made sheets of filo if we are craving crispy, golden pastry. However, if you are really against ultra-processed foods (which we are 95 per cent of the time), then just leave the pastry off. If you are using the ready-made filo, do use refrigerated rather than frozen, as it is less fragile. Unwrap it and use the sheets asap, keeping any leftovers tightly wrapped – they dry out quickly and break. I've kept this vegetarian, but there is nothing to say you couldn't add a layer of the Simple Beef Stew or the Lamb Ragu (see pages 114 and 124).

Bring a large pan of water to the boil. Add the celeriac or swede and boil for 20–30 minutes, or until soft.

Heat 1½ tablespoons of the ghee or butter in a large frying pan over a medium heat. Add the onion, season, and fry for 8–10 minutes until soft. Add the garlic and fry for a couple of minutes before adding half the mushrooms, half the herbs and some seasoning. Turn the heat up and fry the mushrooms over a sizzling heat to drive away the water.

Tip into a bowl and fry the other half of the mushrooms and herbs, adding a little more of the ghee or butter if necessary.

When the celeriac is done, drain it and put into a food processor, or use a stick blender or masher, with the milk, ricotta and seasoning, to taste, then blitz or mash. Once smooth, transfer this mixture to a large ovenproof dish. Tip the mushrooms over the top.

Heat the oven to 220°C/200°C fan (425°F), Gas Mark 7.

Pat the peppers dry on kitchen paper and then add to the blender, or use the stick blender, to blitz them into a purée, adding salt to taste. Pour this layer over the mushrooms. Now crumble or grate the cheese over this layer; it doesn't have to be neat, little mouthfuls of molten cheese are wonderful!

Unwrap the filo and gently crumple 2 sheets, then place over the pie. Gently brush these with half the melted butter, then add a further 2 sheets, aiming to get height in the centre. Brush these with the remaining butter and scatter over the seeds.

Bake the pie for 15–17 minutes or until the pastry is golden brown and crisp. Serve straight away.

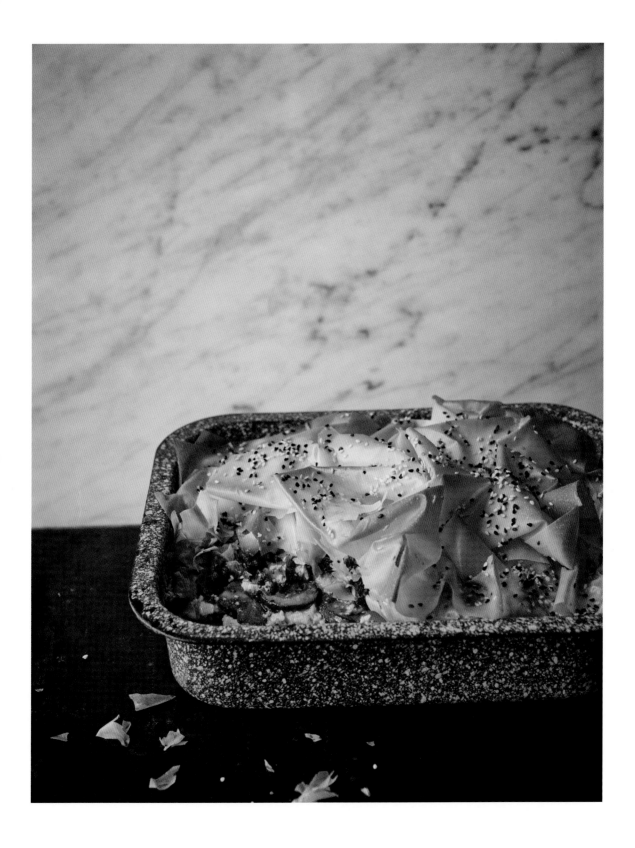

CORONATION CHICKEN

Serves 6

6 tablespoons extra-virgin olive oil
6 spring onions, finely chopped
2–3 teaspoons curry powder (I like 3), or more to taste
a little fresh hot chilli (to taste), chopped, or a pinch of chilli flakes, or more to taste
100g (3½oz) mayonnaise
100g (3½oz) 10% fat Greek yoghurt
500g (1lb 2oz) cooked chicken, torn into bite-sized pieces
4 celery sticks, roughly chopped
1 red pepper, cored, deseeded and diced
150g (5½oz) cherry tomatoes, halved
juice of 1 small lemon
1 head of soft lettuce
salt and pepper

To serve (optional)
lemon wedges
coriander or parsley, torn

PER SERVING: NET CARBS 4g | FIBRE 1.7g
PROTEIN 28g | FAT 32g | 421kcal

This is my low-carb version that is still fit for a king. Rather than smother the chicken in a heavy sauce, I prefer to splash a lighter version over the top. It's great for using up leftover cooked chicken or turkey, or for parties, as it can be prepared in advance, leaving just the salad to make on the day. Do choose a good curry powder; it will make all the difference.

If you don't have cooked chicken, poach chicken breasts in a pan of boiling water, making sure they are covered, for 20–30 minutes, or until they are cooked through and no pink can be seen when you cut into the thickest part. Leave to cool in the water for 15 minutes, then drain and tear into shreds.

Heat 2 tablespoons of the oil in a medium frying pan and fry the spring onions over a medium heat for 5–7 minutes until soft. Season and add the curry powder and chilli, then stir through. Remove from the heat and allow to cool.

Mix the mayonnaise and yoghurt together in a bowl and stir in the cooled onions. Taste the mixture and season as necessary with more salt or spices.

Toss the chicken, celery, pepper and tomatoes in a bowl with the remaining olive oil, lemon juice and a little seasoning. Tear the leaves of the lettuce, discarding the hard core and any damaged leaves, and place on a large serving dish. Tip the chicken mixture over the lettuce and finish by splashing the creamy mixture on top. Garnish as you like with lemon, herbs or extra chilli and serve straight away.

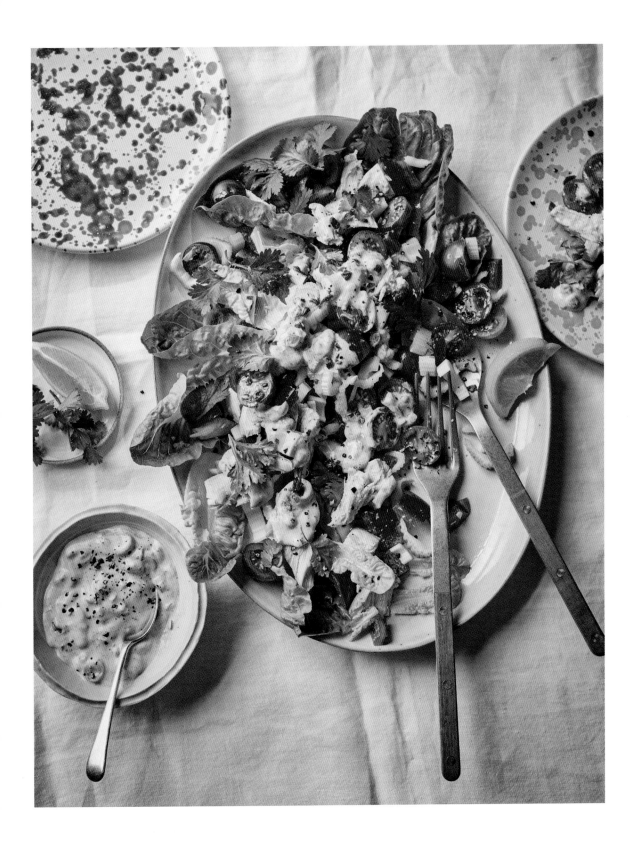

PULLED PORK

Serves 8

1 tablespoon chicken fat or
    dripping or extra-virgin olive oil
2kg (4lb 8oz) meaty pork ribs
1 onion, roughly chopped
4 garlic cloves
2 sprigs of rosemary
4 tablespoons bourbon or brandy
    (optional)
400g (14oz) can chopped
    tomatoes
1 tablespoon cider vinegar or red
    wine vinegar
1 tablespoon tomato purée
1 litre (1¾ pints) chicken or
    vegetable stock
salt and pepper

For the spice mix
1 teaspoon smoked paprika
½ teaspoon ground cumin
½ teaspoon ground cinnamon
1 teaspoon chipotle chilli flakes or
    chipotle paste

PER SERVING: NET CARBS 3g | FIBRE 1g
PROTEIN 47g | FAT 39g | 572kcal

This is a great one for family lunches. Since you end up tearing the meat to shreds, you don't need to spend hours cooking a pork shoulder. Instead, I like to use meaty pork ribs, which have plenty of flavour and fall apart easily after a slow cook. This is my adaptation and will probably offend proper barbecue fanatics but we love it in our family and we know it isn't loaded with sugar! Chipotle (pronounced chi-pot-ley) is a smoked variety of chilli that adds a rich, smoky flavour. If you can't find it, use chipotle paste or chilli flakes instead. It will take 2 to 3 hours in the oven or over the hob or 8 hours in a slow cooker.

Heat the fat in a large frying pan (with a lid) or casserole dish or slow-cooker pan over a medium high heat. Working in batches, brown the pork for 10–15 minutes on all sides. Season the pork in the pan. Remove the meat from the pan and place in a bowl. Place the pan over a medium heat and cook the onion and garlic in the fat for 8–10 minutes until soft.

If you are using the oven, heat it now to 200°C/180°C fan (400°F), Gas Mark 6.

Put the pork back in the pan and scatter over the spice mix and rosemary, moving the pieces around to evenly distribute it. Let it cook for a couple of minutes and, when it is sizzling hot, add the bourbon or brandy, if using. After a minute or 2, this will have mostly evaporated, cleaning the delicious browning from the bottom of the pan.

Now add the tomatoes. Fill the can with warm water and add this, too, along with the vinegar, tomato purée and chicken stock. Stir through.

Bring the mixture up to the boil and put on the lid on. Reduce the heat to low and leave to gently simmer on the hob or in the oven for 2½–3 hours, stirring a couple of times, or until the meat falls from the bone. Alternatively set your slow-cooker to 8 hours on low. Keep an eye on the pork to make sure there is enough liquid to stop it catching.

Using a slotted spoon, scoop out the meat and put in a bowl to cool. Let the sauce settle in the pan off the heat. Spoon off any obvious fat from the pan. Place the pan over a medium–high heat and let it reduce for a few minutes, until you have a sticky, rich sauce.

Discard any bones and any obvious gristle. Using forks, pull the steaks apart and when the sauce has reduced, put the pulled pork back into the pan and thoroughly reheat. Taste the sauce and adjust the seasoning and chilli to your liking. Serve with the sides opposite or the Coleslaw on page 161 and Roasties on page 166.

PULLED PORK SLIDERS

We love a dash of spicy heat in our version of sliders, the small American buns filled with barbecued meat. This can come from our own homemade version of Hot Chilli Sauce or use Frank's Original Red-Hot Sauce, which doesn't have added sugar. We use Jen Unwin's coleslaw, but even the crunch of just shredded raw red cabbage with a little salt is delicious. Pictured with the Smoky Mary Shots overleaf.

Serves 8

8 Sliders (see Rustic Rolls on page 175)
½ quantity Pulled Pork (see opposite), hot
150g (5½oz) gherkins, sliced
200g (7oz) Coleslaw alla Unwin (see page 161)
60g (2¼oz) Hot Chilli Sauce (see page 67) or Frank's Original Red-Hot Sauce
80g (2¾oz) Avo Non-mayo (see page 72) or homemade mayonnaise (see page 65)

PER SERVING: NET CARBS 11g | FIBRE 5g
PROTEIN 32g | FAT 52g | 662kcal

Open up the Sliders and fill with hot Pulled Pork topped with the rest of the ingredients. Tuck in and enjoy!

SMOKY MARY SHOTS

This is our son Giorgio's twist on a Bloody Mary. Apart from the natural sugars in the tomatoes, a Bloody Mary is one of the few sugar-free cocktails available and worth remembering the next time you are at the bar! We often blend a can of Italian plum tomatoes in place of the tomato juice.

Makes 2 highball glasses or 8 shots

100ml (3½fl oz) chilli or regular vodka
400ml (14fl oz) tomato juice or blended canned tomatoes
2 teaspoons lemon juice
¼ teaspoon smoked or unsmoked paprika
few drops of Tabasco sauce
few drops of Worcestershire sauce
½ teaspoon celery salt
pinch of salt
freshly ground black pepper
ice
2 small celery sticks, to garnish

PER SERVING (OF 2):
NET CARBS 7g | FIBRE 1g | PROTEIN 2g | FAT 0g | 150kcal
PER SERVING (OF 8):
NET CARBS 2g | FIBRE 0g | PROTEIN 0g | FAT 0g | 38kcal

Mix all the ingredients together in a jug and adjust the seasoning to taste. Fill 2 glasses with ice, pour over the cocktail and garnish with the celery just before serving.

If you don't serve straight away, it will keep in the refrigerator for up to 1 day.

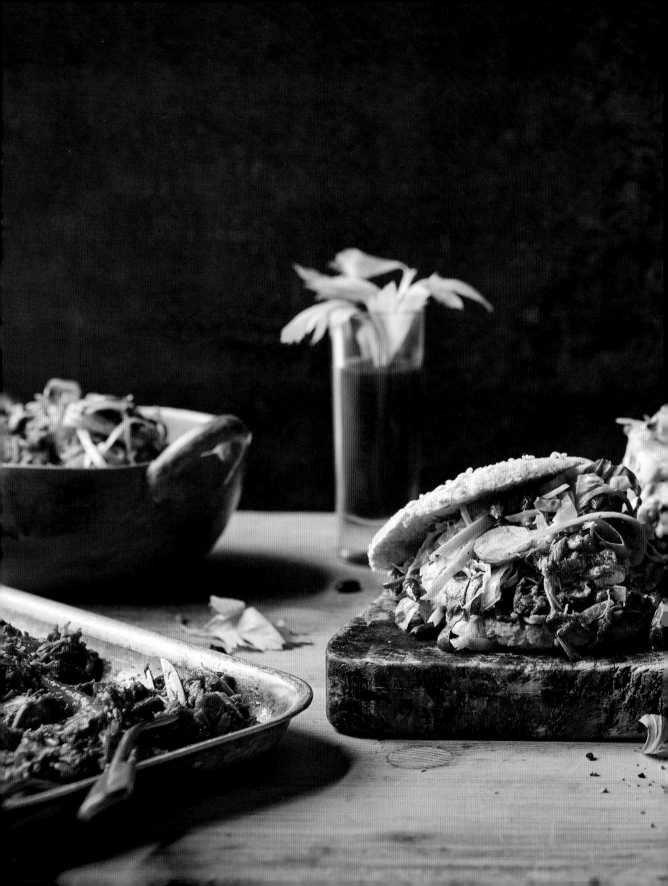

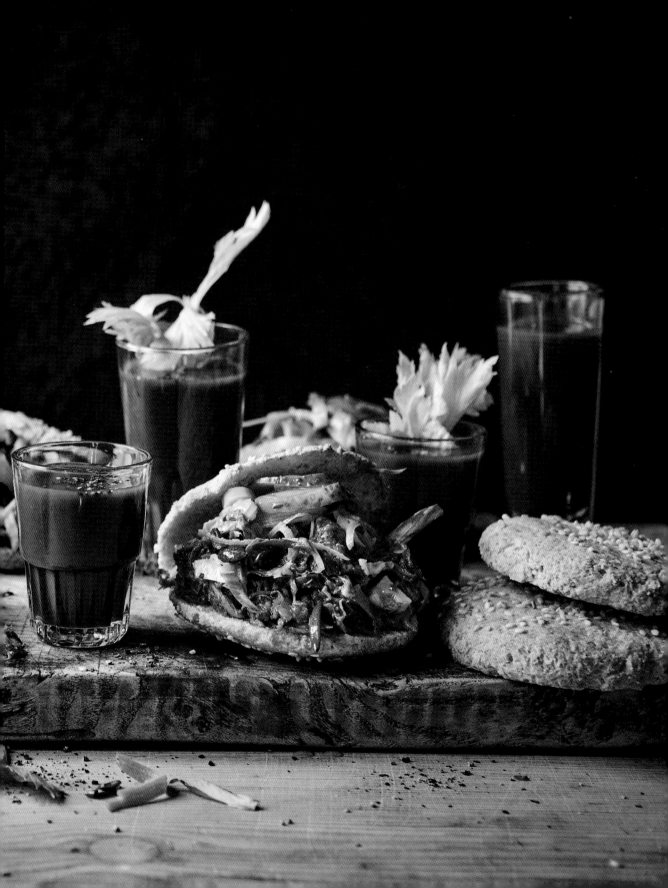

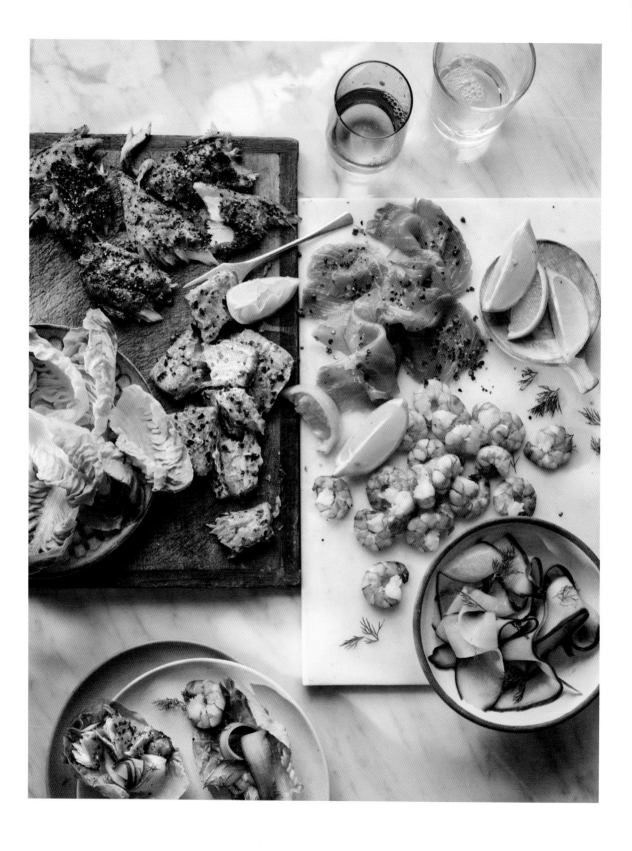

SEAFOOD SMORGASBORD

Serves 8

½ long cucumber, pared into
    ribbons, using a swivel peeler
3 tablespoons red wine vinegar
400g (14oz) smoked or poached
    salmon, or a mixture
400g (14oz) smoked, peppered
    mackerel
400g (14oz) cooked and peeled
    prawns
1 lemon, cut into 8 wedges
2 baby gem lettuces
salt and pepper

PER SERVING: NET CARBS 3g | FIBRE 1g
PROTEIN 31g | FAT 14g | 268kcal

I love a wooden platter. I have about 20 wooden chopping boards of various shapes and sizes, and I know I drive my family mad when I'm on holiday and can't resist trying to pack yet another one into my suitcase. Food just looks great served on sharing platters in the middle of the table. The only recipes to make from scratch here are a healthier version of Marie-Rose sauce and pickled cucumber; the rest can be tipped out of packets while your guests aren't watching. Finish with a few lemon wedges and you have an amazing platter of seafood ready for a feast. These quantities are for a substantial starter portion, so do add more fish and perhaps some hard-boiled eggs for a main course. For fun, and to get a party going, serve Smoky Mary (see page 147) in shot glasses on the side.

Put the cucumber into a bowl with the vinegar and some seasoning. Leave to marinate for a few minutes or up to 3 hours. Serve in a small dish with a little of the vinegar or drain and put straight onto the board.

When you're ready to serve, assemble the remaining ingredients on the platter.

MARIE-ROSE SAUCE

Serves 8

100g (3½oz) shop-bought or
    homemade mayonnaise (see
    page 65)
100g (3½oz) 10% fat Greek yoghurt
4 tablespoons tomato purée
2 tablespoons lemon juice, or
    more to taste
1 teaspoon Worcestershire sauce
½ teaspoon cayenne pepper or
    chilli powder, or more to taste
salt and pepper

PER SERVING: NET CARBS 1g | FIBRE 0g
PROTEIN 1g | FAT 11g | 105kcal

Apparently, Fanny Craddock invented this sauce, but as it was served to the divers who helped rescue the sunken ship, the Marie-Rose, it was renamed. If you are avoiding ultra-processed foods, make your own mayonnaise: see the recipe on page 65 or use the Avo Non-mayo on page 72. This is my version of this famous sauce.

Mix the ingredients together in a small bowl. Adjust the heat, lemon and seasoning to your liking. Serve straight away or keep in the fridge for up to 3 days.

SEAFOOD AND NDUJA STEW

Serves 8

4 tablespoons extra-virgin olive oil

80–100g (2¾–3½oz) nduja

4 garlic cloves, lightly crushed

2 onions, finely sliced

500g (1lb 2oz) fresh, or frozen and defrosted, raw calamari (squid), cleaned and cut into 1cm (½-inch) rings

200ml (7fl oz) dry white wine

3 × 400g (14oz) cans Italian plum tomatoes, chopped

1 tablespoon tomato purée

250g (9oz) clams or mussels or a mixture

1–2 teaspoons smoked paprika (optional)

500g (1lb 2oz) monkfish, cod or coley or other firm fish, cut into bite-sized pieces

250g (9oz) raw prawns, heads left intact, shells and black veins removed

small handful of parsley, leaves and stems roughly chopped

salt and pepper

PER SERVING: NET CARBS 9g | FIBRE 3g
PROTEIN 28g | FAT 14g | 275kcal

Seafood is excellent on a low-carb diet as it is high in protein for satiety and low in carbs. Nduja (pronounced nn-du-ya) is from Calabria in Southern Italy and has become famous only over the past few years. It is a spicy, spreadable salami that has a warm heat and just makes everything it touches a little more interesting. Used here for an instant hit of garlic, chilli and umami, it is a brilliant background for the fish without overwhelming them. Versions of nduja can alter, so do taste yours to see if it is very spicy or salty, and adjust the amount you use accordingly. You can always add more later or add smoked paprika to taste. Serve on its own in bowls or with cauli-rice and low-carb bread on the side for mopping up the sauce. If buying frozen calamari, do read the label carefully; the cooked variety simply needs warming in the sauce rather than a slow-cook.

Heat the olive oil and 80g (2¾oz) of the nduja in a frying pan (with a lid) over a medium heat for a few minutes, bashing the nduja with a wooden spoon to break it up. Add the garlic and onions, then continue to cook for around 10 minutes, stirring to prevent it burning, until the onion is soft.

Add the calamari to the pan and let it cook until the water is released from the calamari, about 10 minutes. When the calamari has a 'bouncy' appearance, add the wine and allow this to evaporate for 5 minutes. Add the tomatoes and the purée and bring the stew to a bubbling heat. Then lower the heat and simmer for at least 1½ hours, partially covered, or until the calamari is soft.

Keep the clams or mussels in the fridge until you are ready to use them. Generally they are purged and cleaned when you buy them but to be sure, put them into a bowl of cold water and stir them through. Leave them for 20–30 minutes in a cool place (the fridge if your kitchen isn't cool), stirring a few times to encourage them to release any grit. Pick over them, discarding any that remain open once tapped. Pull any fuzzy beards off the mussels. Discard any shellfish with broken shells. Drain and use straight away.

Taste the stew and add more nduja or smoked paprika for spice or salt and pepper. The stew can be cooled and kept for 1–2 days at this point, if it makes entertaining easier. Reheat until bubbling before continuing.

Just before serving, drop the monkfish, prawns and mussels, if using, into the hot stew with the lid on and continue to cook for around 10 minutes, or until the fish is cooked through, the prawns are pink and the clams or mussels have opened (discard any that haven't). Serve straight away with the parsley scattered over.

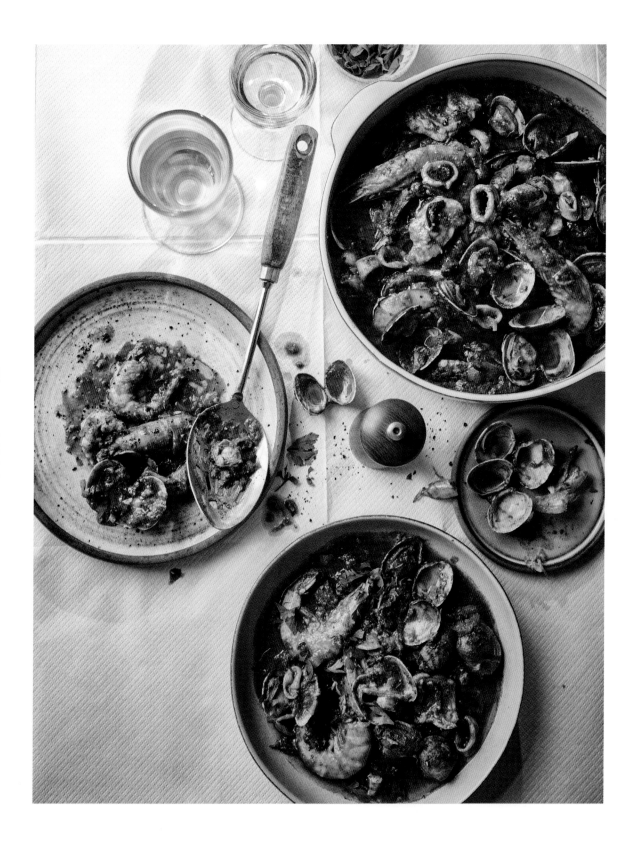

LOW-CARB SWAP

FAST-FOOD FRENCH FRIES

35G CARBS

VS

CRUNCHY AUBERGINE CHIPS (PAGE 157)

4G CARBS

There are so many ways to eat a diverse range of vegetables – whether it is buttered greens, roasted Mediterranean vegetables, a rainbow of salad in a bowl, cauli-rice or celeriac mash – that I never crave potatoes or rice. Jenny and I like to say 'fill your plate with vegetables', which tends to ensure you're eating abundantly but without the carbs and calories of starchy foods.

Enjoying some vegetables before you eat something starchy has been shown to lower the impact of the starchy food on your blood glucose. This is because the fibre in the vegetables causes the starch to be digested more slowly. Our modern society seems to be cottoning onto this now, yet the ancient Romans always started a meal with antipasti!

By eating vegetables with olive oil or butter you enable your body to access the fat-soluble vitamins, so don't shy away from adding a drizzle of healthy fat.

VEGETABLE
SIDES & SALADS

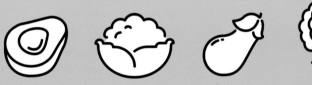

CAULI-RICE

Serves 4

approx. 400g (14oz) cauliflower
   (including stalk and leaves)
3 tablespoons extra-virgin olive
   oil, ghee, butter, coconut oil,
   chicken fat or beef dripping
1 onion or 5 spring onions, finely
   chopped
1 level teaspoon salt
100ml (3½fl oz) warm water
freshly ground black pepper

**PER SERVING CAULI-RICE OR SPICY
CAULI-RICE:** NET CARBS 4g | FIBRE 2g
PROTEIN 2g | FAT 10g | 121kcal

PER SERVING ROAST CAULI-RICE:
NET CARBS 5g | FIBRE 3g | PROTEIN 3g
FAT 10g | 127kcal

To avoid the spikes of glucose in your bloodstream from eating any kind of rice, switch to cauli-rice. It takes just minutes to prepare and you can add endless flavour possibilities if you stir-fry it. It keeps well, once cooked, in the refrigerator for up to 3 days (or in the freezer for up to 3 months), so leftovers are quick to reheat. You can also use broccoli or sprouts in the same way. Once riced, the vegetables expand in volume; you need to allow around 100g (3½oz) raw cauli-rice per person.

This is delicious any time you would have eaten conventional rice or as a meal with a couple of fried eggs.

Cut the head of the cauliflower into large florets and roughly chop the stalk and leaves. Put one-third of the cauliflower into a food-processor and pulse until finely chopped (it will resemble large grains of rice), making sure you don't end up with a purée. Tip the cauliflower into a bowl and repeat with the remaining two-thirds. If you don't have a food-processor, coarsely grate the florets and stalk and finely chop the leaves.

Heat the fat in a wok or large frying pan (with a lid). Add the onion and fry over a medium heat for 7 minutes or until soft. Add the cauliflower rice, season and stir through. Add the warm water, cover and leave to cook over a low heat for around 8 minutes or until just soft, stirring occasionally to make sure it doesn't stick to the bottom.

Taste and add seasoning as necessary. If any water remains, remove the lid and allow it to evaporate over the heat while you stir it.

Serve straight away or leave to cool and reheat later. The rice will keep, cooked and cooled, in the refrigerator for up to 4 days. It can be reheated in a pan with a lid or in the microwave.

Spicy Cauli-rice
For a spicy kick, stir a pinch of chilli flakes and a teaspoon of ground cumin through the onions after they are cooked. Finish with plenty of chopped fresh coriander.

Roast Cauli-rice
Roasting cauli-rice gives a nutty, lightly toasted flavour. Heat the oven to 220°C/200°C fan (425°F), Gas Mark 7. Put the cauliflower rice on a baking tray lined with baking paper then toss with the oil, salt and pepper, making sure everything is coated. Roast for 20 minutes, stirring halfway, until lightly browned and just soft.

CRUNCHY AUBERGINE CHIPS

Serves 6

35g (1¼oz) whole white or black chia seeds

75g (2¾oz) ground almonds

1 large aubergine, courgette or pepper (approx. 325g/11½oz)

35g (1¼oz) Parmesan cheese, finely grated

¼ hot chilli powder or cayenne pepper

1 teaspoon salt

plenty of freshly ground black pepper

2 eggs

2 tablespoons extra-virgin olive oil

PER SERVING: NET CARBS 4g | FIBRE 5g
PROTEIN 8g | FAT 17g | 209kcal

We love anything made with a breadcrumbed crust; however, that isn't so good if you are watching your weight. By experimenting with chia seeds, I am so excited to have created these crunchy chips with a soft centre and loads of flavour. They even keep in the refrigerator or freezer and reheat brilliantly, so do make them in batches. They are great for serving with a quickly cooked steak (see page 102) or with the Sliders on page 147. I have given options for adding heat but you could use finely chopped rosemary or smoked paprika for flavour instead of the chilli or cayenne; the possibilities are endless. They are also great made in an air-fryer or with courgettes and peppers instead of aubergine.

Heat the oven to 220°C/200°C fan (425°F), Gas Mark 7. Line a baking tray with baking paper.

If you have a mini food processor, very briefly grind together the chia seeds and almonds, so you are left with partially fine and partially whole seeds.

Cut the aubergine or courgette in half widthways and trim the stalk. Cut into chips around 1.5cm (⅝ inch) wide. If using peppers, core, deseed and cut into chip-width strips.

In a shallow bowl, use a spoon to stir together the chia, almonds and Parmesan with the chilli or cayenne, salt and black pepper. Crack the eggs in another bowl and beat.

Use tongs to dip the chips, a few at a time, into the egg, then drop them into the chia mixture and use a spoon to toss them around to make sure they are coated all over. With a little care you should be able to do this process without adding excess egg to the dry mix. Use your fingers to gently pick them out of the bowl and lay them on the lined tray. Bake for 18–20 minutes or until lightly browned and crisp, turning the tray halfway through if they are not cooking evenly.

Serve straight away, drizzled or brushed with the oil. Alternatively, allow the chips to cool and store in the refrigerator for 2 days. Reheat in the oven before serving.

MARIETTA'S GREEN BEANS AND CHERRY TOMATOES

Serves 4

500g (1lb 2oz) green, runner or flat beans, topped and tailed and stringed if necessary, large beans halved
3 tablespoons extra-virgin olive oil
100g (3½oz) cherry tomatoes, halved
2 garlic cloves, roughly chopped
pinch of chilli flakes
salt and pepper

PER SERVING: NET CARBS 6g | FIBRE 4g
PROTEIN 3g | FAT 10g | 132kcal

This is Giancarlo's mother, Marietta's, way of cooking green beans that turns a humble vegetable into something savoury and delicious. The beans should be soft and not squeaky. They are great with meat, fish and eggs and keep well for 3 days in the refrigerator. You can also make this with frozen beans.

Bring a saucepan of water to the boil. Add the beans and cook for around 10–15 minutes, or until soft and flexible. Drain when ready.

Meanwhile, heat the oil in a frying pan over a medium heat. Add the tomatoes, garlic, chilli and seasoning and fry for 5 minutes, or until the tomatoes have softened and started to create a rough sauce. Add the beans and stir them gently through. Taste for seasoning. Serve in a warm bowl.

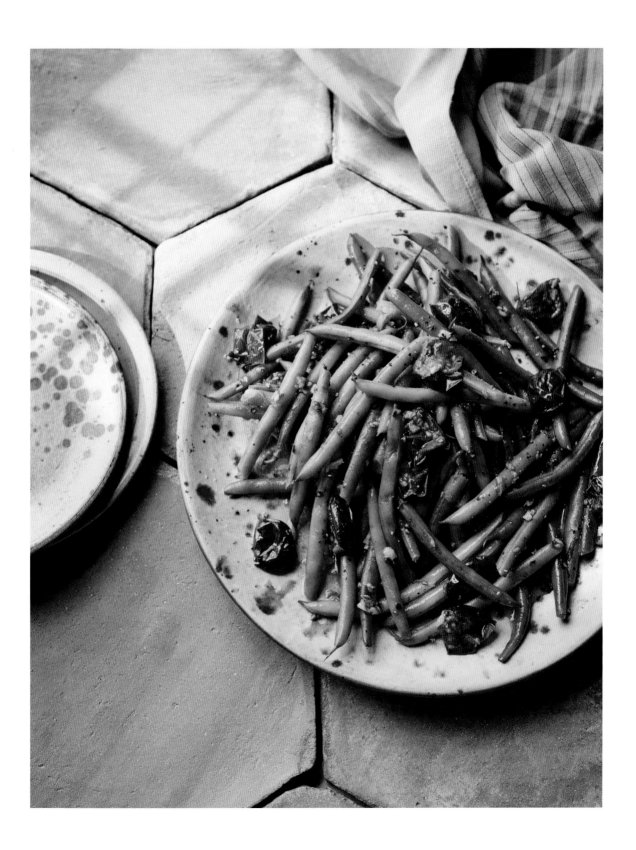

STIR-FRIED SPROUTS
WITH ONION, BACON AND WALNUTS

Serves 6

75g (2½oz) whole walnuts or pecans
1 tablespoon extra-virgin olive oil
25g (1oz) butter
1 onion, finely chopped
4 thick smoked streaky bacon
    rashers, cut into strips
500g (1lb 2oz) Brussels sprouts,
    shredded
100ml (3½fl oz) water
salt and pepper

PER SERVING: NET CARBS 6g
FIBRE 3g | PROTEIN 7g
FAT 19g | 220kcal

These sprouts are so tasty that they make a good meal on their own or with a couple of fried eggs, and by shredding them you can tell the sprout-haters it's cabbage! Traditional chestnuts are higher in carbs than other nuts, so I have replaced them with soaked walnuts or pecans to offer a creamy texture and golden colour. You can fry the bacon and onion in advance and have them ready in a pan. I never peel or trim sprouts unless the leaves are damaged or brown; I shred them in a food processor or cut them by hand, and keep them in an airtight container in the refrigerator until I need them.

Put the nuts into a small bowl with just-boiled water to soak.

Heat the oil and butter in a large frying pan or wok (with a lid) over a medium heat. Fry the onion and bacon together for 10–12 minutes, until the bacon is cooked and the onions are translucent. Season lightly.

Drain the nuts, then add to the pan with the sprouts and water. Stir-fry them over a high heat for 5 minutes to mingle the flavours together. Cover with the lid, increase the heat to medium and cook for 5 minutes, shaking the pan occasionally.

Remove the lid and check that they are just soft. If not, fry for a little longer. Taste and adjust the seasoning as necessary. Serve straight away, keep warm or allow them to cool and reheat just before serving.

COLESLAW ALLA UNWIN

Serves 6

3 spring onions, bulbs and green
  parts, finely chopped
1 teaspoon cider vinegar or red
  wine vinegar
50g (1¾oz) pine nuts or chopped
  walnuts or pumpkin seeds
2 gem lettuce hearts (approx.
  250g/9oz), shredded
150g (5½oz) cauliflower, Brussels
  sprouts or firm white, purple or
  green cabbage, finely shredded
1 large carrot, coarsely grated

For the mustard dressing
1 tablespoon cider vinegar or
  lemon juice
2 teaspoons Dijon mustard
4 tablespoon extra-virgin olive oil
2 tablespoons crème fraîche or
  10% fat Greek yoghurt (optional)
salt and pepper

**PER SERVING FOR THE MUSTARD
DRESSING:** NET CARBS 4g | FIBRE 2g
PROTEIN 2g | FAT 15g | 158kcal

**PER SERVING FOR THE CREAMY
DRESSING:** NET CARBS 4g | FIBRE 2g
PROTEIN 2g | FAT 17g | 174kcal

This is Dr Jen Unwin's recipe for a quick, crunchy coleslaw. You can use any member of the cabbage family to make up the volume. We sometimes add a green chilli for a kick or throw in 25g (1oz) chopped coriander for a variation. And if we want it creamy, we add crème fraîche or Greek yoghurt.

Variety is key to getting a diverse range of nutrients in your food, so the more colourful, the better. If you have a food processor, this takes very little time, but you can also use a mandoline or sharp knife. I have collected gadgets over the years and love my Vietnamese carrot shredder and my mother's old cheese slicer; both give quick and interesting cuts to salad vegetables.

Soak the spring onions for 15 minutes in cold water with the vinegar to dilute their strength.

Heat a frying pan over a medium heat and dry-fry the nuts in the pan until lightly browned. Toss them into a large serving bowl.

Combine the dressing ingredients in a bowl, seasoning to taste. Drain the onions and add the remaining ingredients to the salad bowl. Stir the dressing through to combine, making sure the nuts at the bottom join in the fun. Serve straight away.

ICEBERG WEDGES WITH AVOCADO AND KEFIR SALAD CREAM

Serves 6

1 iceberg or other crunchy lettuce (approx. 230g/8oz)
1 avocado, sliced
2 celery sticks, roughly chopped
2 tablespoons extra-virgin olive oil, for drizzling
1 quantity Avo Non-mayo (see page 72) or Green Chilli and Herb Kefir (see page 71)
approx. 10 chives, finely chopped
1 teaspoon pink peppercorns (optional)
salt and pepper

PER SERVING: NET CARBS 3g | FIBRE 3g PROTEIN 2g | FAT 17g | 179kcal

Giancarlo loves the crunch of iceberg lettuce and piles his plate high with this salad. It's great with barbecues and feasts as it doesn't wilt quickly on a buffet table. It can be prepared to the chopped and plated stage a few hours before serving.

Cut the iceberg in half, discarding any damaged outer leaves and the stalk end. Next, cut the halves into further large wedges and into half again. Lay these on a large serving plate in a single layer.

Add the avocado and celery and, just before serving, drizzle over the oil and season with salt and pepper. Splash over either dressing, scatter over the chives and peppercorns, if using, and serve straight away.

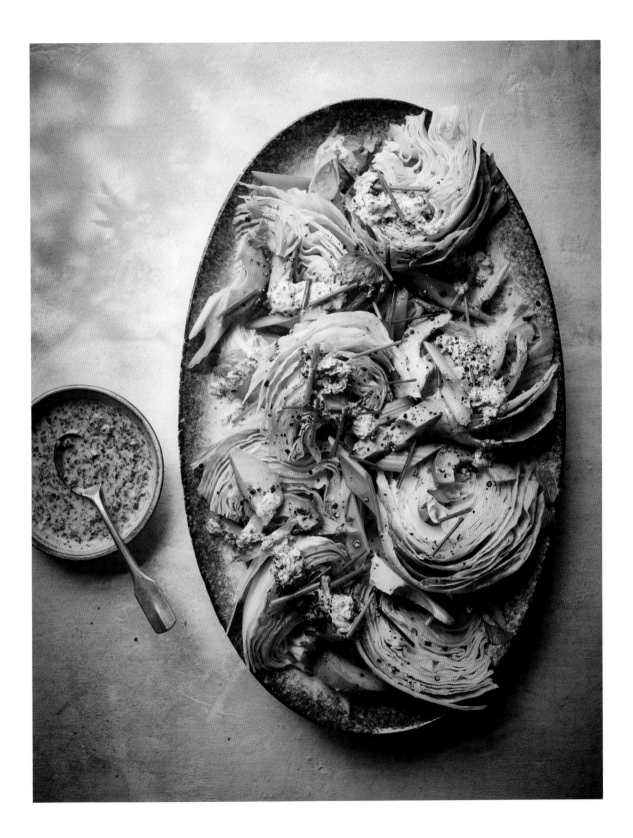

HOMAGE TO DELIA LAYERED SALAD

Serves 6

1 quantity Italian Roast Vegetables
    (see page 167), at room
    temperature
50g (1¾oz) quinoa (optional)
600g (1lb 5oz) cauliflower, riced
    (see page 156)
3 tablespoons extra-virgin olive oil
1 romaine lettuce heart or baby
    gem lettuce
200g (7oz) feta or crumbly goats'
    cheese, cubed
handful of coriander or parsley,
    stems finely chopped and
    leaves roughly chopped
1 teaspoon black onion (nigella)
    seeds
salt and pepper

**For the harissa and lemon
    dressing**
3 tablespoons shop-bought
    harissa paste
3 tablespoons lemon juice
5 tablespoons extra-virgin olive oil

PER SERVING: NET CARBS 19g | FIBRE 7g
PROTEIN 10g | FAT 32g | 416kcal

PER SERVING WITH QUINOA:
NET CARBS 24g | FIBRE 8g
PROTEIN 11g | FAT 32g | 446kcal

This is my favourite salad in *Delia's Summer Collection* cookbook. I've had the pleasure of meeting her and hearing about her passion for teaching the nation to cook, and this is my low-carb version of her salad, in homage to her illustrious career. I have used cauliflower in place of couscous and cheated on the sauce. Add the quinoa if you are not going keto, as it helps to bulk up the cauliflower rice and adds a little protein. This makes an excellent light summer lunch or a substantial side dish to roast meats.

Heat the oven to 220°C/200°C fan (425°F), Gas Mark 7. Line a baking tray with baking paper.

Cook the quinoa, if using, according to the instructions on the packet (it normally takes around 20 minutes). You can tell when it's done when the tails of the seeds come away from the centre.

Meanwhile, put the cauliflower rice on the lined tray and dress it with the oil, salt and pepper. Use your hands to toss it together, making sure everything is coated. Roast in the oven for 20 minutes or until lightly browned and just soft.

Make the dressing by mixing the ingredients together, adding seasoning if necessary.

Remove the cauliflower rice and set aside. When the quinoa is done, drain and mix it with the cauliflower on the tray. (I use my hands or a large spoon for this.) Use the baking paper to tip this into a large serving dish. Top with the roasted vegetables.

Roughly chop or tear the lettuce over the vegetables and then add the feta. When you are ready to serve, pour the dressing over the lot and finish with the herbs and onion seeds.

Harissa Paste
If you don't want to use a shop-bought harissa paste, we have a recipe on our website, www.thegoodkitchentable.com

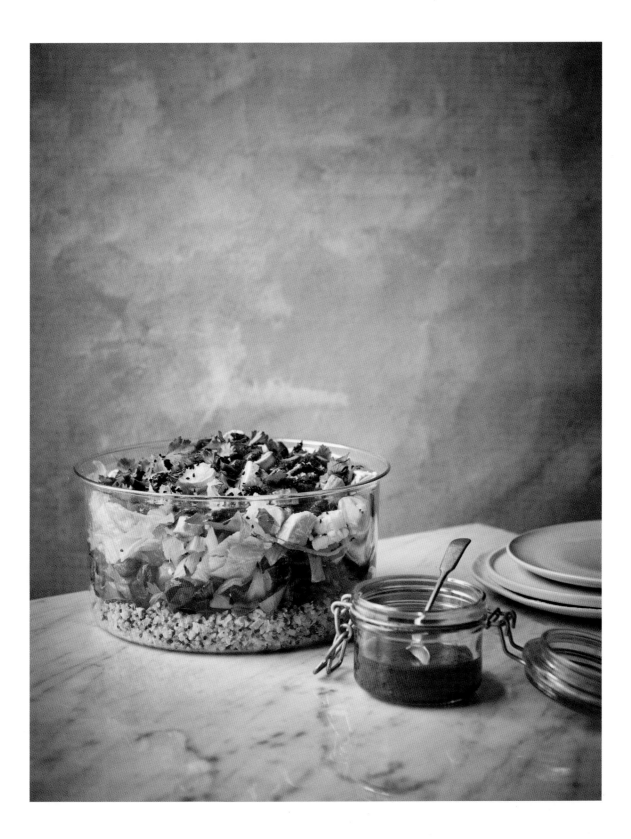

ROASTIES

Serves 6

1kg (2lb 4oz) root vegetables (such as carrots, parsnip, celeriac, swede, radishes, Brussels sprouts or turnips)
1 onion, cut into wedges
5 tablespoons extra-virgin olive oil
4 small sprigs of rosemary
1 teaspoon dried oregano
4 bay leaves
6 large sage leaves, roughly chopped
2 teaspoons fennel seeds
2 fat garlic cloves, unpeeled and crushed
salt and pepper

PER SERVING: NET CARBS 12g
FIBRE 6g | PROTEIN 1g
FAT 12g | 168kcal

We love the jewel-like colours of these roast vegetables, and the flavour from the herbs is fantastic. You won't miss potatoes at all! All of the peelings can be kept in the freezer and used for a homemade stock another day. The roasties are best served straight from the oven, but can be prepared up to the point just before cooking and kept in a bowl in the refrigerator for up to a day. Leftovers can be reheated under foil in the oven until piping hot. See photo on page 138.

Heat the oven to 220°C/200°C fan (425°F) Gas Mark 7.

Scrub and cut the carrots and parsnips, if using, into wedges that are about 3cm (1¼ inches) at the fattest end. Peel and dice the swede and/or celeriac into 3cm (1¼-inch) dice and cut the sprouts in half.

Toss the vegetables and onion in a bowl with the oil, seasoning, herbs and spices. Spread them out on a baking tray and roast for 30 minutes or until cooked through.

Serve straight away or keep warm, loosely covered, for up to 1 hour.

ITALIAN ROAST VEGETABLES

Serves 4

5 tablespoons extra-virgin olive oil

1 small aubergine, cut into 1cm (½-inch) slices

1 small courgette, cut into 1cm (½-inch) slices

1 red or yellow pepper, cored, deseeded and cut into finger-width strips

1 onion, cut into finger-width wedges

2 garlic cloves, unpeeled and lightly crushed

2 sprigs of rosemary, thyme or sage

salt and pepper

PER SERVING: NET CARBS 11g | FIBRE 4g | PROTEIN 2g | FAT 17g | 215kcal

This is our staple recipe for roasting vegetables Italian-style; we swap in what's in the refrigerator and garden. It makes enough for 6, as I always like to have a bowl in the refrigerator for adding to salads, frittatas, soups, etc. These are great as an accompaniment to meat, fish and poached eggs, as a base for pasta sauces or with a soft, creamy burrata or buffalo mozzarella and a scattering of basil.

Always tuck the herbs under the vegetables to give flavour and stop them burning, and space the vegetables out so that they evenly roast rather than steam in a pile.

Heat the oven to 220°C/200°C fan (425°F), Gas Mark 7. Grease a baking tray with a little of the olive oil.

Put the vegetables into a bowl with the remaining olive oil, a large pinch of salt and some pepper, then toss to combine. You need the oil to stop the vegetables burning, so don't be tempted to be mean with it! Evenly spread the vegetables over the tray in one layer (you may have to use 2 trays). Add the garlic and tuck the herbs under the vegetables to stop them burning. Bake for 25–30 minutes or until lightly browned and cooked through.

Transfer the vegetables to a serving dish and serve hot or at room temperature. Any leftovers will keep for a couple of days in the refrigerator.

CREAMY MASH

Serves 4

400g (14oz) low-carb vegetable(s) (such as cauliflower, celeriac, pumpkin, swede, Brussels sprouts or broccoli), roughly chopped into even-sized pieces

25g (1oz) salted butter or extra-virgin olive oil, plus extra to serve

25–75ml (1–2½fl oz) full-fat cows' milk, cream, crème fraîche or water

½ teaspoon freshly grated nutmeg or 1 tablespoon finely chopped chives, parsley or basil (optional)

salt and pepper

PER SERVING OF SPROUT MASH:
NET CARBS 4g | FIBRE 3g | PROTEIN 3g
FAT 7g | 97kcal

PER SERVING OF CAULI OR BROCCOLI MASH: NET CARBS 4g | FIBRE 2g |
PROTEIN 2g | FAT 7g | 88kcal

PER SERVING OF SWEDE MASH:
NET CARBS 3g | FIBRE 1g | PROTEIN 1g
FAT 6g | 67kcal

PER SERVING OF PUMPKIN MASH:
NET CARBS 3g | FIBRE 1g | PROTEIN 1g
FAT 7g | 68kcal

PER SERVING OF CELERIAC MASH:
NET CARBS 3g | FIBRE 4g | PROTEIN 2g
FAT 6g | 84kcal

Non-starchy vegetables are perfect for making creamy mash with a fraction of the carbs of potato. Celeriac mash, for example, contains 4g (1/8oz) carbs per serving compared to potato mash at 24g. Celeriac is good with meat as well as fish; while cauliflower, sprouts and swede are better with meat, sausages and eggs. Pumpkin is also good and lower carb than butternut squash. By using the leaves and stalk of the brassicas you get a lot more mash. Cut the stalks into smaller pieces than the rest of the vegetables and cook these first. Add the leaves last to ensure even cooking.

Vegetable mash can be made with a potato masher, but a food processor or stick blender gives the creamy texture that we all love. This recipe works for all vegetables but as some are more absorbent than others, you will have to alter the milk quantity. Add nutmeg or herbs for extra flavour if you are feeling adventurous!

Steam or boil the vegetables until tender when pierced with a sharp knife, then drain well.

Blend with the remaining ingredients in a food processor or with a stick blender until you have a soft, smooth mash. Taste and adjust the seasoning as necessary.

Serve straight away or keep warm until you are ready to serve. The mash keeps well in the refrigerator for up to 4 days and freezes for up to 3 months.

ONION, CHEESE AND MUSTARD MASH

Serves 4

15g (½oz) butter
1 tablespoon extra-virgin olive oil
100ml (3½fl oz) warm water
1 onion or leek, finely chopped
1 quantity of Creamy Mash (see opposite)
25g (1oz) Parmesan cheese, finely grated
1–2 teaspoons Dijon or Coleman's mustard
salt and pepper

PER SERVING: NET CARBS 7g | FIBRE 2g
PROTEIN 5g | FAT 11g | 141kcal

For extra flavour, add onions, cheese and mustard to your cooked vegetable before mashing.

Melt the butter into the oil with the warm water in a large saucepan over a low heat. Add the onion or leek with a little seasoning and steam-fry for about 10 minutes, stirring frequently until soft. Add the Creamy Mash, cheese and mustard and stir through. Taste and adjust the seasoning and mustard heat as you like.

Bread must be one of the most popular comfort foods. My favourite way to eat it is buttered toast with Marmite and a cup of Earl Grey tea. Readers always tell me that bread is one of the hardest foods to give up when you cut back carbs. However, with my low-carb baking recipes you will be pleased to know that bread, muffins and even cake can be enjoyed on a low-carb diet. The seeded crackers are a great substitution for wheat based ones; we love them to pack them up for long journeys or to eat with cheese at the end of a meal.

The low-carb dough is incredibly versatile – it can be used to create rolls, sliders, pizza bases and flatbreads. I like to prepare a double quantity, divide it up into the various shapes and sizes and then freeze, so I have a freezer full of different options.

A few of my top low-carb baking tips are overleaf.

BAKE & DIVIDE

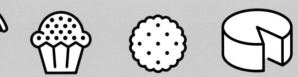

Low-carb baking

Do look at the various recipes in this chapter, the time they take, whether they contain gluten or not, their carb counts and purpose and decide which is right for you. For further free-from bread recipes, see www.thegoodkitchentable.com.

I love bread, but I have seen what it does to my blood glucose levels (see page 23). Since I am metabolically healthy, my body can restore itself quickly, so I don't rule it out completely but choose not to eat it every day, or I will put on weight. Giancarlo, on the other hand, is gluten intolerant and has poor insulin sensitivity, so he has to be more careful with bread. The low-carb, gluten-free recipes are ideal for him.

Gluten – Gluten is the name for the proteins gliadin and glutenin found in grains such as wheat, spelt, rye, emmer, einkorn and barley. Giancarlo and our son Giorgio tested positive for gluten intolerance several years ago, so I have been creating gluten-free recipes for years. Some people with mild gluten intolerance find that there isn't a problem with wholemeal ancient grains such as spelt and rye, but we are all different! Do read Dr David Unwin's thoughts about gluten on page 22 and for further notes and references, see www.thegoodkitchentable.com.

Here are a few hero ingredients that will help your lower-carb baking:

Oats – These are naturally gluten-free nutritious grains; however, they are often milled in factories that use gluten, so read the packet carefully. Oats are broken down and sold in many ways: the oat kernel without the hull (outer shell) is called a groat, which can be boiled or chopped, hence steel-cut oats. Any product made from the groats such as oatmeal, quick or instant oats are high in carbs, and the finer they are milled, the quicker they will raise glucose levels. A recent product to the low-carb market is oat fibre, which is the ground hull and is insoluble fibre. There are two kinds; a white, fluffy oat fibre, which I prefer, or a brown more powdery version which is heavier and sometimes needs more water added to it. It adds bulk but almost no carbs, so is perfect for low-carb baking. However, it is not a straight replacement for wheat flour. Oat bran is the outermost part of the groat and contains soluble and insoluble fibre. It is high in protein and low in carbs and fat. It has a nutty, slightly sweet flavour.

Psyllium husks – Found in health food shops and online, these are a form of fibre from the ovata plant, which work as a binder and help baked goods rise. Buy blonde psyllium husks for golden bread and try to find the husks rather than the expensive powdered psyllium. This does work, but can produce a purple-coloured bread. One word of warning: the psyllium husk needs to cool down after it is baked, as it firms up as it cools, so no nibbling on the bread before it is at room temperature, or you will find a soggy dough.

Coconut flour – A fine powder that is very absorbent, so use in small quantities. It helps bind but also offers a natural sweetness to bread and pastry.

Mozzarella – Its job is to melt between the ingredients, holding them together and then to set firm on cooling. It leaves a mild, savoury taste rather than a cheesy one. It's fine to use the inexpensive pizza mozzarella or the cows' milk one in a bag in the recipes in this chapter. Freeze any that is not used.

Chia seeds – A popular, versatile seed from South America, chia seeds come in black or white colours and swell on contact with liquid, making them ideal for binding in low-carb baking. Although tasteless, they add bulk, protein and fibre to our food.

Mixed seeds – Seeds such as sunflower, pumpkin and sesame contain protein and fat and are nutritious. They can be used whole for texture or ground into flour. Like everything we eat, enjoy a diverse selection of seeds.

Ground almonds – The main substitute for wheat flour in low-carb baking is finely ground blanched almonds, also known as almond flour. You can grind your own almonds with or without the skin, the only difference is the colour. Almonds are low in carbs, have little flavour and add body and fat to baked goods.

Linseed – Also known as flaxseed, it is cheaper to buy the whole seed and grind your own. The golden-coloured seeds produce a golden bread, and the darker seeds give a dark rye-style bread, but the taste is the same. Grind the seeds twice in a small high-speed food processor to make flour. Grinding it twice helps to prevent a slimy texture to the bread. Linseed also helps to keep you regular and offers a good supply of omega-3 fat.

Butter – Usually it doesn't matter if it is salted or unsalted, but try to always go for one made with milk from grass-fed cows.

Eggs – It doesn't matter if they are medium or large, but either extreme, i.e. very small or very large, might affect the result. I have added the size if it is important.

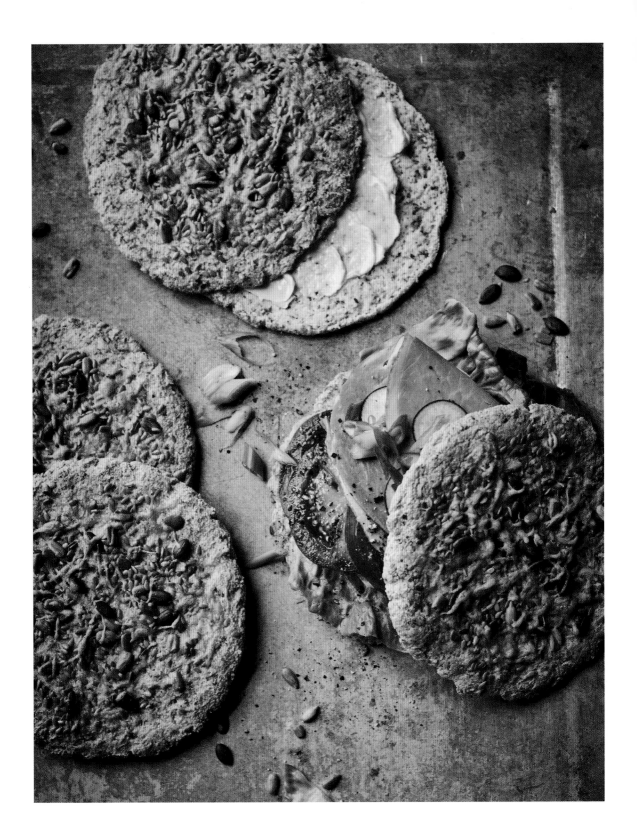

RUSTIC ROLLS

Makes 4 Rustic Rolls or 8 Sliders

oil, for greasing
150g (5½oz) ground almonds
1 heaped teaspoon baking powder
10g (¼oz) psyllium husks
25g (1oz) oat fibre or oat bran
1 teaspoon salt
175ml (6fl oz) cold water
3 eggs
4 teaspoons seeds, to decorate
   (optional)

PER ROLL: NET CARBS 6g | FIBRE 5g
PROTEIN 13g | FAT 25g | 311kcal

PER ROLL WITH HERB AND CHEESE:
NET CARBS 7g | FIBRE 6g | PROTEIN 15g
FAT 27g | 338kcal

PER ROLL WITH BACON: NET CARBS 6g
FIBRE 6g | PROTEIN 16g | FAT 28g |
349kcal

PER SLIDER: NET CARBS 3g | FIBRE 3g
PROTEIN 6g | FAT 13g | 159kcal

Every time I write a new low-carb book, I use the opportunity to perfect my bread recipe. As the years have passed, new products have entered the market and new discoveries in methods arrive. Oat fibre, available online and at some health shops, has revolutionized keto dough, making it light and airy, particularly if you use the white, fluffy, light version. If you can't find it, use oat bran instead.

There is no kneading or rising time here, so this recipe is quick. The large rolls are filling, and so are perfect to have with soup or filled with low-carb ingredients for a portable lunch. Each one is large and filling, so sometimes we find that one split between us is plenty, or you can make the Sliders, which use the same dough divided into 8 small rolls.

Heat the oven to 220°C/200°C fan (425°F), Gas Mark 7 and grease a baking tray with a little oil.

Use a large metal spoon to mix all the dry ingredients together in a large mixing bowl. Add the cold water, then crack the eggs into the bowl and stir everything together with a large spoon. Stir in any additional flavours to the dough, if using, (see overleaf) until it is well combined.

Now the dough can be used to make pizza, rolls or sliders.

To make Rustic Rolls
Using lightly-oiled hands, divide the dough into 4 and shape each piece into a flattened circle about 12cm (4 ¾ inches) wide and 2cm (¾ inch) thick. Place on a prepared baking tray, spaced about 4cm (1½ inches) apart. Scatter over the seeds, if using. Bake for 15 minutes or until golden brown and firm to the touch.

Remove from the oven and transfer to a cooling rack. Serve straight away or leave to cool and store in a container in the refrigerator for up to 3 days or freeze for up to 3 months. Use a serrated knife to carefully slice them in half before using.

RUSTIC ROLLS CONTINUED

To make Sliders

Using lightly-oiled hands, divide the dough into 8 and shape each piece into a roll. Place on a prepared baking tray, spaced about 4cm (1½ inches) apart. Scatter over the seeds, if using, pushing them in gently, and bake for 15 minutes or until golden brown and firm to the touch.

Remove from the oven and transfer to a cooling rack. Serve straight away or leave to cool and store in a container in the refrigerator for up to 3 days or freeze for up to 3 months.

Additional flavours

Herb and cheese – add 25g (1oz) finely grated Parmesan cheese and 4 teaspoons dried oregano to the dough

Bacon – cook 4 rashers of bacon and cut into pea-sized pieces, then add to the dough

CRACKERS

Makes approx. 36

30g (1oz) milled black or white chia seeds
6 tablespoons water
125g (4½oz) ground almonds
10g (¼oz) Parmesan cheese, finely grated
1 teaspoon salt

Optional additions
5g (⅛oz) finely chopped rosemary
1 tablespoon black onion (nigella) seeds or caraway seeds
1 tablespoon cumin seeds

PER CRACKER: NET CARBS 0g
FIBRE 1g | PROTEIN 1g | FAT 2g | 27kcal

I love this simple recipe to make crunchy crackers. They are plain and perfect with cheese, or try embellishing them with seeds or herbs for looks and flavour; they are slightly addictive, so do keep them out of sight! White chia give a paler colour, black seeds give a speckled appearance, but either colour works fine. If yours aren't milled, use a small, high-speed food processor to do the job or soak them in the water first for 15 minutes.

Cut 2 pieces of baking paper the same size as a large baking tray, approx. 30 × 40cm (12 × 16 inches).

Mix the ingredients together in a mixing bowl with a spoon to form a smooth, thick dough.

Heat the oven to 180°C/160°C fan (350°F), Gas Mark 4.

Put the dough into the centre of one piece of the baking paper on a work surface. Put the other sheet on top. Use your hands to push the mixture down and then use a rolling pin to evenly roll out the dough to a thickness of 3mm (⅛ inch). Use a knife to move some of the dough around, if needed, and to neaten the edges so you have a rectangle that almost fills the tray. Slowly peel away the top sheet of paper and make sure there aren't any holes. If there are, gently push the mixture together with a finger dipped in water (to stop it sticking to you).

Use a cook's knife or wiggly pasta cutter to score lines in the dough to form crackers around 5 × 5cm (2 × 2 inches). Now transfer this base sheet to the baking tray and bake in the oven for 15–17 minutes, or until golden brown.

Remove the crackers from the oven and slide the paper from the tray onto the work surface. Now break up the crackers along the scored lines. Leave them to cool for a few minutes, then transfer to a cooling rack.

The crackers will keep in an airtight container for up to 3 days or in the refrigerator for a week. If they do soften, re-bake them in a hot oven for a few minutes. You can also freeze them.

LOW-CARB PIZZA OR FLATBREAD

**Makes 4 pizzas
(approx. 18cm/7 inches)**

olive oil, for greasing
1 quantity Rustic Rolls dough
   (see page 175)

For the tomato sauce
160g (5¾oz) tomato passata or
   canned whole Italian plum
   tomatoes
1 teaspoon dried oregano
¼–½ teaspoon salt
freshly ground black pepper

For the toppings
125g (4½oz) mozzarella cheese,
   drained
150g (5½oz) salami slices
Kalamata olives, pitted and halved
slices of red chilli

To serve
1 tablespoon extra-virgin olive oil
handful of basil leaves

PER PIZZA: NET CARBS 7g
FIBRE 14g | PROTEIN 29g
FAT 55g | 681kcal

PER ZA'ATAR FLATBREAD: NET CARBS 5g
FIBRE 13g | PROTEIN 14g
FAT 29g | 372kcal

We all know a good pizza is hard to beat. We love it the world over, as it is one of the most umami-rich (savoury and tasty) foods we can find. However, it is high in carbs – from the base and the tomato sauce – and with the fat from the cheese, is usually highly calorific; so pizza should be a treat, not an everyday food.

Our low-carb pizza is both crisp around the edges and supports the taste of the topping without overwhelming it – and kids love it. As the pizza bases contain almonds and plenty of fibre, they are filling, so you need only a small portion of this delicious food, with a large salad.

Heat the oven to 220°C/200°C fan (425°F) Gas Mark 7. Line 2 oven trays with baking paper and brush with oil.

Divide the dough into 4 pieces and put 2 mounds of the dough on each lined tray. Press and shape each piece with damp hands into a circle about 18cm (7 inches) in diameter and 1cm (½ inch) thick. Bake in the oven for 10 minutes.

Meanwhile, blend all the tomato sauce ingredients together with a stick blender or fork, seasoning to taste.

Remove the trays from the oven and turn the oven up as hot as it will go. At this stage the bases can also be cooled, covered and kept in the refrigerator for 3 days or frozen for 3 months. Defrost before use.

When you are ready to cook, top each one (still on the paper on the tray) with one-quarter of the tomato sauce, leaving a finger-width border around the edge. Tear over the mozzarella and scatter over the toppings.

Bake for 6–8 minutes until the cheese is bubbling and the crust is crisp and browned.

Remove from the oven and serve with a drizzle of olive oil and the leaves scattered over.

Variation: za'atar flatbreads
Make and shape a pizza base according to the recipe above. Before it is cooked, brush over a tablespoon of extra-virgin olive oil and scatter 1 heaped teaspoon of shop-bought or homemade za'atar (see www.thegoodkitchentable.com) over each base. Cook for 12–14 minutes at 220°C/200°C fan (425°F), Gas Mark 7.

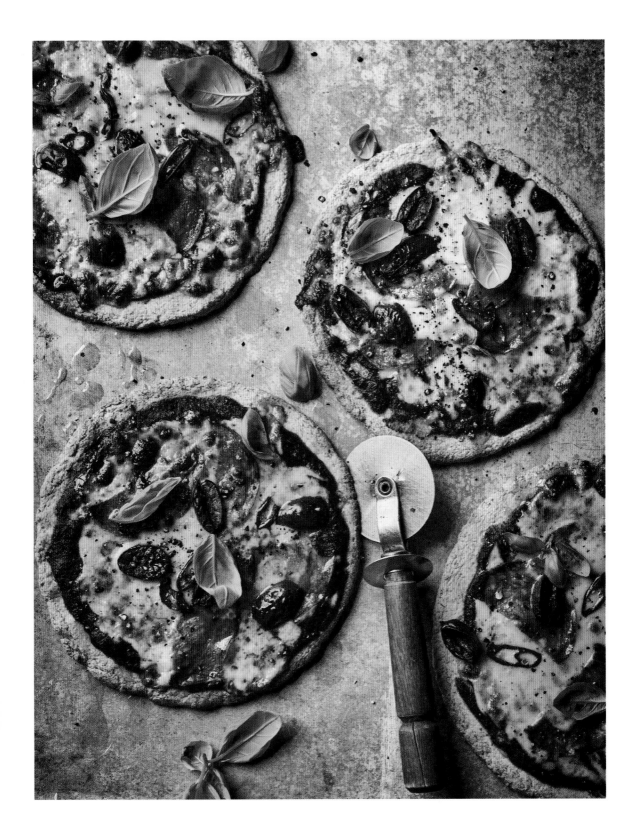

SAUSAGE ROLLS

Makes 16 rolls

6 high-meat content, gluten-free
    sausages (approx. 400g/14oz)
1 egg yolk, beaten, to glaze
1 tablespoon sesame seeds, for
    topping (optional)

For the pastry
150g (5½oz) ground almonds
150g (5½oz) mozzarella cheese,
    coarsely grated
½ teaspoon salt
2 tablespoons brine from the
    mozzarella, or water

PER ROLL: NET CARBS 1g | FIBRE 1g
PROTEIN 5g | FAT 10g | 116kcal

Nutritionist Jenny Phillips asked me to create low-carb sausage rolls for her, as her family has a tradition of eating them at Christmas. She used to peel off the pastry to avoid the gluten, but I am happy to say that this year she can enjoy the whole sausage roll. Do seek out good-quality sausages with no or little added rusk (Italian sausages are good) and make sure you buy a gluten-free variety if you are gluten intolerant. Do use vegetarian sausages if you prefer, but note that the carb quantity will be different.

Cut 2 pieces of baking paper the same size as a large baking tray.

To make the pastry, use a food processor to blend the ingredients together or put the ingredients into a bowl and use a spoon to stir and squeeze them together to form a smooth, thick dough.

Use your hands to gather it into a ball and divide it in half. Gently roll each half into a sausage shape.

Place the dough sausages on one piece of baking paper, about 10cm (4 inches) apart. Lay the other piece of baking paper on top and use a rolling pin to roll the dough sausages into two long, thin rectangles about 12 × 30cm (4½ × 12 inches) long and 3mm (⅛in) thick. You can cut away misshapen pieces and add them in as necessary to make your rectangles. You shouldn't have any leftover dough.

Heat the oven to 200°C/180°C fan (400°F), Gas Mark 6. Peel the skin from the sausages (or simply squeeze the meat out) and lay 3 along the centre of each rectangle. Obviously, some sausages are shorter or fatter than others, so squeeze or stretch the sausage meat accordingly to fit the length. Use the baking paper to lift the pastry from each edge and roll up to cover the sausages. Use a serrated knife to gently cut each roll into 8 pieces, cleaning the knife frequently so it doesn't stick and tear the pastry. Use one of the pieces of baking paper to line the baking tray.

Carefully lift the sausage rolls onto the prepared tray. Brush with the egg yolk and scatter over the sesame seeds, if using. Bake for 20 minutes until the pastry is golden brown.

Remove from the oven and serve the sausage rolls warm or at room temperature. Once cooled they will keep in a sealed container in the refrigerator for up to 3 days or in the freezer for up to 3 months.

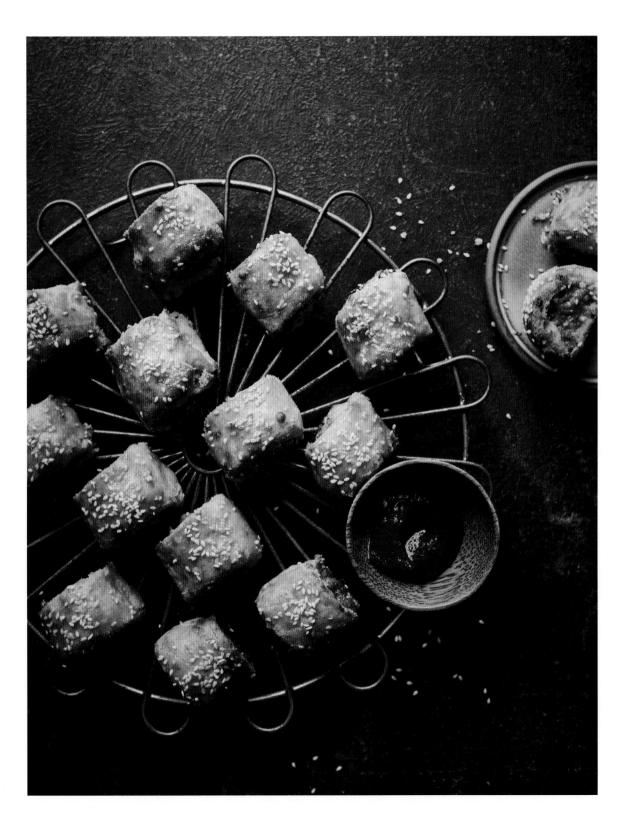

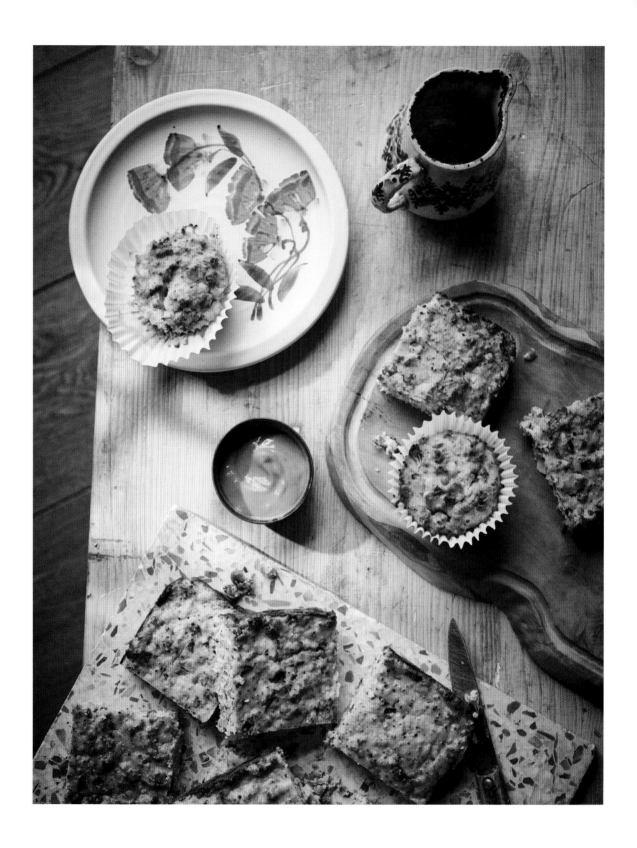

SMOKED CHEESE MUFFINS

Makes 12 muffins or 9 squares

butter, for greasing
4 eggs
200g (7oz) ground almonds
200g (7oz) cottage cheese
35g (1¼ oz) whole chia seeds
50g (1¾oz) smoked or mature
   Cheddar cheese, finely grated,
   plus extra to cover
4 smoked bacon rashers, cooked
   and finely chopped
150g (5½oz) cauliflower or
   broccoli, cut into pea-sized
   pieces
100g (3½oz) peas
8 spring onions, finely chopped
½ teaspoon chopped hot chilli or
   a pinch of chilli flakes
good pinch of salt
plenty of freshly ground black
   pepper

PER MUFFIN: NET CARBS 6g | FIBRE 12g
PROTEIN 15g | FAT 23g | 329kcal
PER SERVING: NET CARBS 7g | FIBRE 16g
PROTEIN 31g | FAT 31g | 438kcal

These are an excellent breakfast on the run or to take on journeys or to work, as they have a good amount of protein in the egg, bacon, cheese and chia and fibre in the vegetables. You may want to microwave a small batch for speed; for a guide, one muffin takes 2 minutes at full power (900W).

Generously grease a 20cm (8inch) square or round cake tin with butter or prepare 12 paper muffin cases in a muffin tray or 12 silicone muffin moulds.

Mix all the ingredients together in a bowl. Heat the oven to 200°C/180°C fan (400°F), Gas Mark 6.

Divide the mixture between 12 muffins case or pour all of it into the baking tray. Put into the oven to bake for 15–20 minutes.

Check the muffins are cooked through by piercing them with a skewer. If it comes out clean, they are done; if it is wet, put them back into the oven for another few minutes.

MINUTE MUFFINS

These muffins are an adaptation of the popular mug cake but with a fraction of the carbs. Using ripe fruit gives flavour, natural sweetness and colour, and do use it in season; strawberries in summer are so much better than forced winter ones. When the fruit is naturally sweet you may find you can omit the honey or sweetener. The muffins can be cooked conventionally in the oven or cooked quickly in minutes in the microwave, which is the more energy efficient option.

STRAWBERRY AND VANILLA

Makes 6 muffins

100g (3½oz) roughly chopped, ripe, soft fruit such as strawberries, raspberries, pear or peach
2 eggs
100g (3½oz) ground almonds
50g (1¾oz) softened butter or coconut oil
½ teaspoon baking powder
2 teaspoons vanilla extract and/or pinch of ground cinnamon
2 teaspoons honey or 1 heaped tablespoon erythritol
100g (3½oz) 10% fat Greek yoghurt, to serve
zest of ½ lemon

PER MUFFIN WITH YOGHURT (WITH HONEY OR ERYTHRITOL):
NET CARBS 8g | FIBRE 2g | PROTEIN 7g | FAT 19g | 215kcal

For oven cooking, prepare a muffin tin with paper cases or use a silicone muffin mould. When using a microwave, I use small coffee cups as muffin moulds, sometimes with paper cases in them. If baking, heat the oven to 200°C/180°C fan (400°F), Gas Mark 6.

Reserve 25g (1oz) chopped fruit for decoration. Mix the remaining ingredients, except the yoghurt, together in a bowl and divide between the moulds.

Microwave the muffins on full power (900W) for 2 minutes, 30 seconds. If they're still wet on top, give further 10 seconds blasts until done. Or, bake them in the oven for 15–20 minutes. Piece with a skewer: if it comes out clean, they are ready; if it is wet, put them back in the oven for another few minutes.

Serve the muffins warm, or cool and decorate with the yoghurt, lemon zest and reserved fruit.

COFFEE AND CHOCOLATE

Makes 6 muffins

2 eggs
80g (2¾oz) ground almonds
½ teaspoon baking powder
2 teaspoons vanilla extract
2 teaspoons honey or 1 tablespoon erythritol (optional)
20g (¾oz) unsweetened cocoa powder
10g (¼oz) dark chocolate drops or dark chocolate, roughly chopped
1 teaspoon instant coffee granules (optional)

PER MUFFIN (WITH HONEY OR ERYTHRITOL):
NET CARBS 13g | FIBRE 7g | PROTEIN 10g | FAT 15g | 243kcal

Follow the instructions on the left to prepare and cook the muffins.

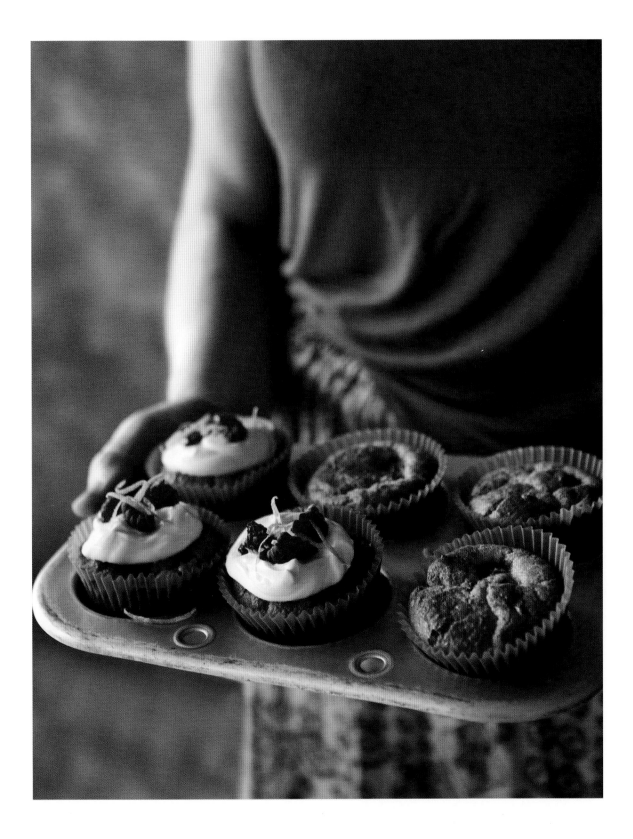

LOW-CARB SWAP

REGULAR BROWNIE

50G CARBS

VS

CHOCOLATE, DATE AND
WALNUT BROWNIE (PAGE 188)

5G CARBS

Yes, it is possible to have low-carb desserts, and they are delicious too! These recipes give you the choice of adding natural sweetness in the form of fruit or using a sweetener such as honey or erythritol.

When divided into small portions the 'carb hit' in these recipes is usually manageable and very low when compared to traditional desserts, which are almost always sugar laden. However, for some diabetics even around 10g carbs per pudding, such as in the Black Forest Gateau, may be enough to trigger sugar cravings. If that sounds like you, then you may be better sticking to lower carb desserts and focusing on the joy of cream for a bit of decadence instead.

If you are opting for a piece of fruit with, or after, a meal, then berries are the lowest carb options. A single banana, for example, will send sugar levels soaring, as will other tropical fruits like mango and pineapple.

DESSERTS & SWEET TREATS

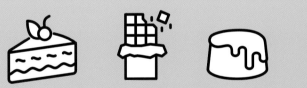

CHOCOLATE, DATE AND WALNUT BROWNIES

Makes 18 brownies

125g (4½oz) walnuts, macadamia
    nuts or pecans, halved
60g (2¼oz) pitted dates, roughly
    chopped or 100g (3½oz)
    erythritol
3 tablespoons hot water (if using
    dates)
125g (4½oz) dark chocolate (at
    least 75% cocoa solids)
75g (2½oz) salted or unsalted
    butter
pinch of salt (if using unsalted
    butter)
100g (3½oz) ground almonds
2 eggs, beaten
½ teaspoon baking powder
2 teaspoons vanilla extract

PER BROWNIE USING DATES:
NET CARBS 5g | FIBRE 2g | PROTEIN 3g
FAT 16g | 174kcal

PER BROWNIE USING ERYTHRITOL:
NET CARBS 2.5g | FIBRE 2g | PROTEIN 3g
FAT 16g | 165kcal

These brownies have minimal sweetness but are packed with flavour. They are also full of fibre from the nuts, chocolate and dates. Toasting nuts brings out their natural oils and gives them oodles of flavour. Smell them as they go into the oven and as they come out and you will see what I mean. If you are keeping your carbs very low, use erythritol instead of dates.

Heat the oven to 220°C/200°C fan (425°F), Gas Mark 7.

While the oven is warming, put the nuts on a baking tray lined with baking paper and lightly brown in the oven for 6–8 minutes; do watch carefully as they burn easily. Use the paper to shoot the nuts onto a plate to cool. Return the paper to the tin. Turn the oven off and close the door to retain the heat, as you'll use it again later.

Line a 20cm (8-inch) square cake tin or similar-sized ovenproof dish with baking paper. Soak the dates, if using, in the hot water for a couple of minutes. Use a fork to mash them to a purée.

Roughly chop the nuts; each nut should be cut into around 4 pieces.

Reheat the oven to 220°C/200°C fan (425°F), Gas Mark 7.

Place the chocolate and butter in a small heatproof bowl and melt together in the microwave for a couple of minutes. If you don't have a microwave, melt the chocolate and butter in a glass or metal bowl over a pan of simmering water, ensuring the bowl does not touch the water.

Add the date purée or erythritol and stir through. If your butter does not contain salt, add a pinch now. Add the remaining ingredients, including the chopped roasted nuts, and stir through to combine. Spoon the mixture into the prepared tin and bake for about 15 minutes until firm to the touch. Remove from the oven and leave to cool in the tin for 10 minutes or so.

Use the paper to remove the brownies from the tin, then cut into 18 squares. Serve at room temperature on their own or with Greek yoghurt or whipped cream and a dash of vanilla extract.

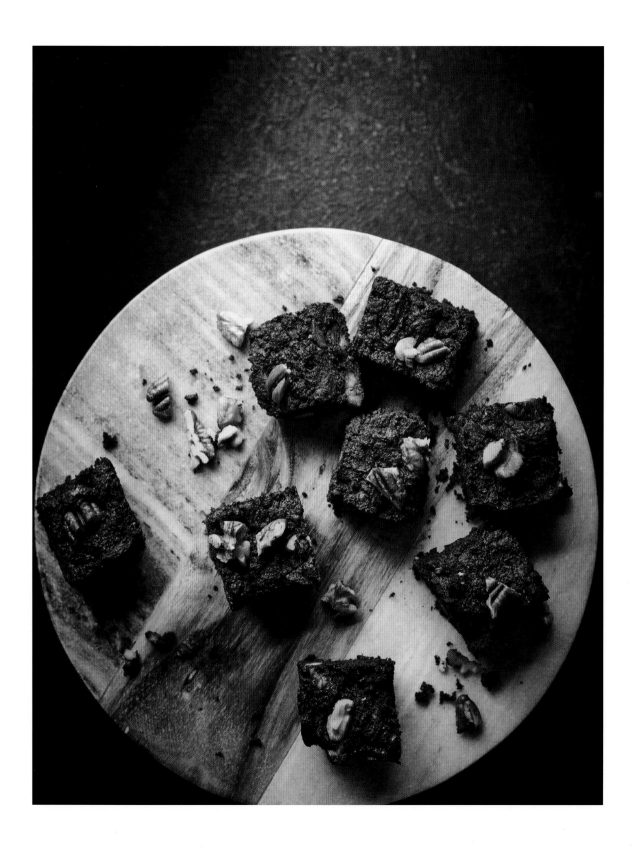

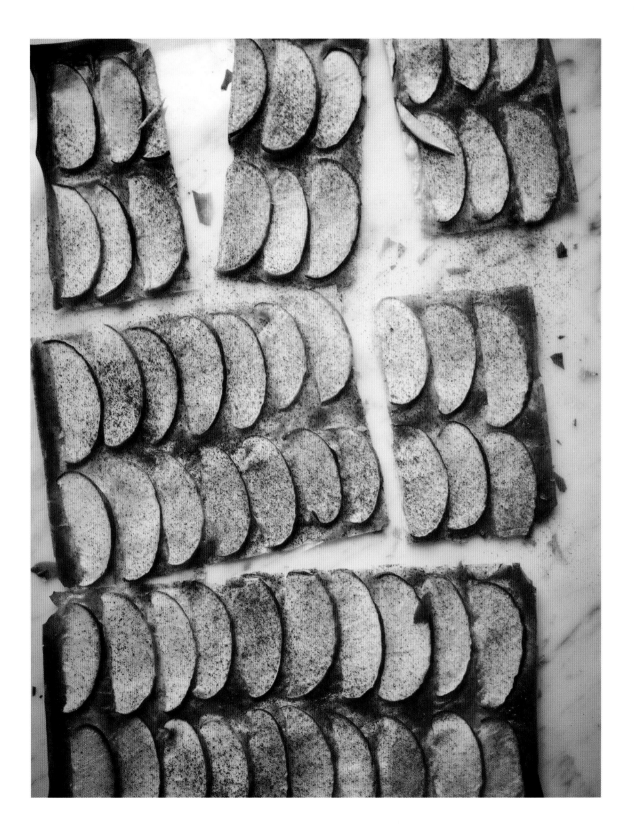

CINNAMON APPLE TART

Serves 6

25g (1oz) salted butter
1 tablespoon honey or 2
   tablespoons erythritol
1 teaspoon vanilla
2 sheets of filo pastry
3 apples, cored and thinly sliced
1 heaped teaspoon ground
   cinnamon

PER SERVING WITH HONEY:
NET CARBS 21g | FIBRE 2g | PROTEIN 2g
FAT 4g | 129kcal

PER SERVING WITH ERYTHRITOL:
NET CARBS 19g | FIBRE 2g | PROTEIN 2g
FAT 4g | 118kcal

The most delicious smell emanates from your oven when this is being prepared. It's winter, Christmas, comfort food and apple heaven in one aroma!

Heat the oven to 220°C/200°C fan (425°F), Gas Mark 7.

Melt the butter with the honey or erythritol and vanilla in a small bowl in the microwave or the oven. Set aside.

Line a baking tray large enough to hold a sheet of filo with baking paper. Unravel the sheets of filo pastry (wrap and freeze the rest for another day) and lay one on the tray. Brush the pastry with a thin coating of the butter mixture. Lay the next sheet on top and brush it again with the butter.

Now lay the apple slices on the pastry, just touching one another. They should cover almost all the pastry, leaving a small border around the outside. Brush with the remaining butter. If you run out of butter (it happens if you are generous!) just make up a little more. Dust with cinnamon and put into the oven for 12 minutes or until brown. If the tart starts to brown too much around the edges before the apple is cooked, fold the foil over the edges to stop this. Serve straight away or leave to cool to room temperature, it's delicious both ways!

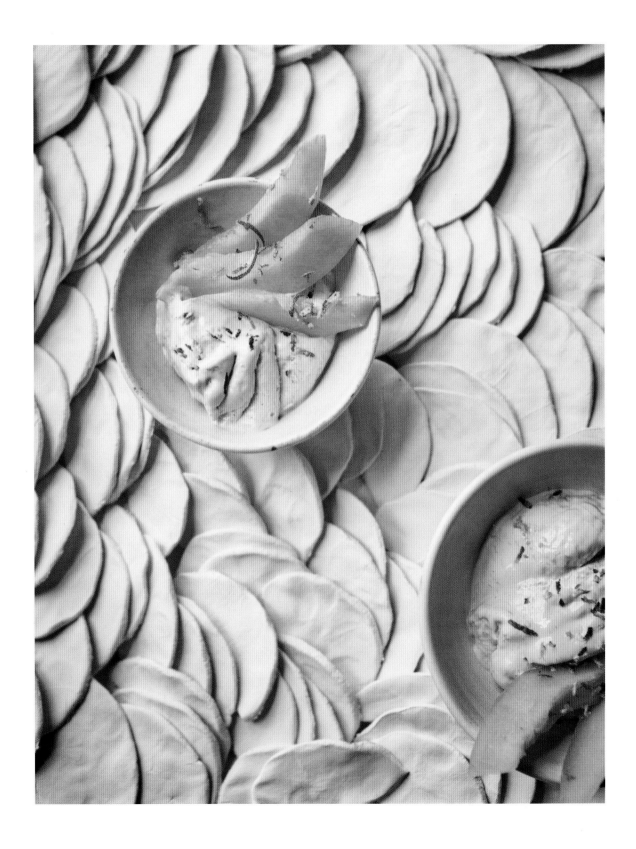

MANGO ICE CREAM

The smaller Alfonso mangoes are perfect for this dish, and they are packed with perfumed flavour. The larger variety simply don't carry the flavour. Don't worry if your mango chopping isn't up to scratch, as the whole lot will be blitzed anyway. If you can't find good mangoes, use the same amount of frozen raspberries instead.

Serves 6

approx. 200g (7oz) ripe Alfonso mango flesh, chopped into 1cm (½-inch) dice
250g (9oz) mascarpone
1 teaspoon vanilla extract

PER SERVING:
NET CARBS 6g | FIBRE 1g | PROTEIN 2g | FAT 19g | 198kcal

Chill 6 small glasses or bowls in the refrigerator or freezer. Line a tray with baking paper.

Spread the mango flesh over the lined tray; try to separate the cubes, so that they don't freeze as one piece. Place in the freezer for at least 2 hours, depending on your freezer, until frozen.

Just before you are ready to eat the ice cream, remove the fruit from the freezer and immediately place in a food processor with the mascarpone and vanilla extract. Blend just enough to break up the fruit, but don't overwhip it or it will melt. (If it melts, call it a smoothie!)

Divide the ice cream between the 6 chilled glasses or bowls and serve straight away.

MELON AND LIME

Lime seems to bring any fruit to life and on melon it is sublime. This is so ridiculously simple but it is such as lovely combination. This is wonderful on its own or with the Mango ice cream on the side.

Serves 6

1kg (2lb 4oz) cantaloupe melon
1 lime

PER SERVING:
NET CARBS 12g | FIBRE 2g | PROTEIN 1g | FAT 0g | 56kcal

Cut the melon into wedges and arrange on a plate. Grate the lime zest over it and serve.

PEACH AND HAZELNUT TART

Serves 10

400g (14oz) peaches, nectarines,
    apricots or berries, stoned and
    finely sliced
200ml (7fl oz) whipping cream
1 teaspoon vanilla extract
3 tablespoons Amaretto, brandy
    or rum (optional)

For the pastry

150g (5½oz) blanched or skin-on
    hazelnuts or other nuts
1 tablespoon honey or 1 heaped
    tablespoon erythritol
100g (3½oz) butter, softened and
    cut into small cubes
40g (1½oz) coconut flour
finely grated zest of ½ orange or
    1 small lemon (optional)
1 teaspoon vanilla extract
1 egg

**PER SERVING WITH AMARETTO AND
HONEY:** NET CARBS 8g | FIBRE 3g |
PROTEIN 3g | FAT 19g | 226kcal

**PER SERVING WITH AMARETTO AND
ERYTHRITOL:** NET CARBS 7g | FIBRE 7g |
PROTEIN 3g | FAT 19g | 221kcal

This stunning dessert is a great choice, even when living a low-carb lifestyle. Use berries or canned apricots, or a mixture of them both if fresh stone fruits aren't in season. This toasted hazelnut pastry is naturally sweetened with orange zest, so it positively bursts with flavour.

Heat the oven to 220°C/200°C fan (425°F) Gas Mark 7.

Roast the nuts on a baking tray for 8–10 minutes or until golden brown, giving the tray a shake halfway. If the nuts have skins, when done, tip them onto a tea towel and fold it over the nuts. Rub the tea towel over the nuts to loosen the skins. Pick out the nuts and put them into a shallow bowl to cool. Turn the oven off and close the door to retain the heat.

Cut a circle of baking paper about 4cm (1½ inches) larger than a 22cm (8½-inch) tart tin. Tear off another piece bigger than this so that you can roll the pastry between them.

If making the pastry by hand, roughly chop the nuts to a texture of sand and gravel, then mix with the remaining pastry ingredients in a bowl with a spoon. Alternatively, blitz the nuts and remaining ingredients briefly in a food processor until just combined. You may need to push the mixture down with a spatula a couple of times.

Reheat the oven, this time to 190°C/170°C fan (375°F), Gas Mark 5.

Place the pastry between the 2 pieces of baking paper and roll out, using the circle as a guide and bearing in mind that you need the pastry to come up the sides of the tin by 1.5cm (⅝ inch). Peel off the larger piece then turn the tart tin over the circle. Put your hand underneath the paper and invert it into the tin. Push the pastry down into the edges and up the sides a little. Be fussy now and make sure the pastry is evenly up the sides and thick enough to hold its shape once cooking. Prick a few holes in the pastry base with a fork to stop it rising. Bake for 12–15 minutes or until firm to the touch and golden brown all over.

Remove the pastry from the oven and let it sit in the tin for 10 minutes to firm up. Then, use the paper to lift it carefully on to a cooling rack. I like to serve it in the paper.

While the tart cools, slice the peaches. Whip the cream with the vanilla and Amaretto, brandy or rum, if using, until it forms soft peaks, then chill in the fridge.

As soon as the pastry has cooled to room temperature, transfer it to a flat serving plate. Spoon the whipped cream into the pastry case and even out with the back of the spoon. Top with the sliced fruits and berries. Serve straight away or chill for up to a day in the refrigerator.

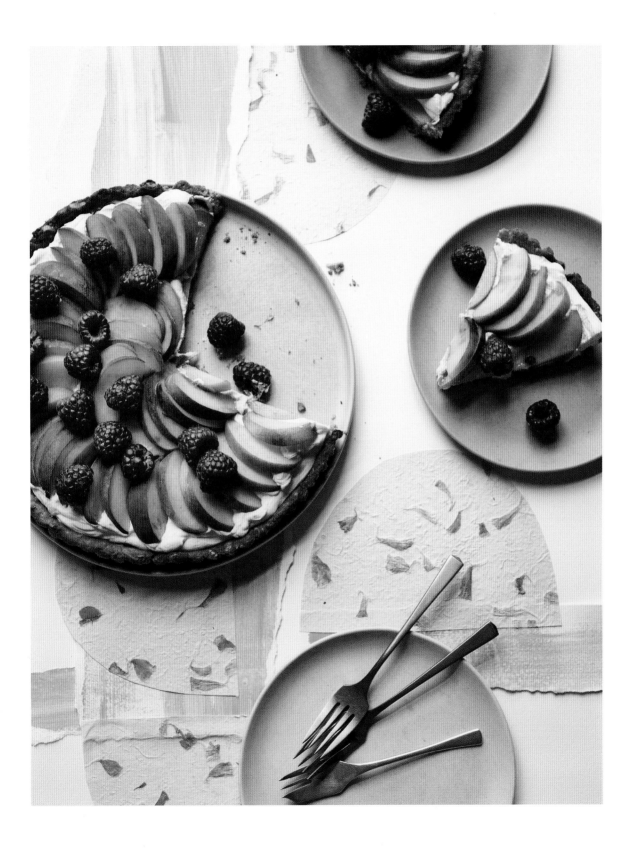

BLACK FOREST GATEAU

Serves 12

For the filling
35g (1¼oz) dried sour cherries
250g (9oz) fresh or 200g (7oz)
    frozen pitted cherries
3 tablespoons Kirsch or Amaretto
25g (1oz) dark chocolate (at least
    75% cocoa solids)

For the sponge
225g (8oz) ground almonds
75g (2¾oz) unsweetened powder
1 heaped tablespoon baking
    powder
1 tablespoon vanilla extract
6 medium eggs
75g (2¾oz) butter, softened
4 teaspoons honey or 2
    tablespoons erythritol
2 tablespoons Kirsch or Amaretto

For the cream
250ml (9fl oz) whipping or double
    cream
1 tablespoon honey
2 teaspoons vanilla extract

PER SERVING WITH HONEY: NET CARBS
13g | FIBRE 3g | PROTEIN 7g | FAT 21g |
271kcal

PER SERVING WITH ERYTHRITOL: NET
CARBS 10g | FIBRE 3g | PROTEIN 6g |
FAT 21g | 261kcal

Some of us remember when this was the Dessert of the Day in the 1970's. Good versions had the distinctive black cherry flavour from sour cherries and Kirsch, which is what we have here, however the sugar is reduced to a few teaspoons of honey and almonds replace white flour. It is a delicious showstopper of a cake and still low in carbs compared to the original recipes, so go ahead and enjoy a slice for a celebration.

Measure enough baking paper to line 2 cake tins, approximately 19cm (7½ inches) in diameter. Wet the paper, scrunch it up, then flatten and use it to line the cake tins.

Place the sour cherries in a small bowl and pour over enough very hot water to just cover them. Leave them to soak while you make the sponge. Pick out the 12 prettiest fresh cherries and set aside for the decoration.Pit the rest of fresh cherries and put into a separate bowl with 1 tablespoon of the Kirsch or Amaretto to infuse.

Heat the oven to 200°C/180°C fan (400°F), Gas Mark 6.

Beat the sponge ingredients together in a bowl until smooth, then transfer to the paper-lined tins, pushing the mixture into the corners of the tins, then flatten the tops with a spatula. Bake in the oven for 8–10 minutes or until the sponge feels firm to the touch and a toothpick inserted into the middle of the cakes comes out clean.

As soon as the sponge is cooked, remove from the oven and leave to cool for 5 minutes. Carefully turn out onto a cooling rack and pierce the cakes with a thin skewer or toothpick. Dilute the remaining 2 tablespoons of Kirsch with 2 tablespoons of cold water and pour this evenly over the sponges. Leave for 20 minutes to cool.

Drain both types of cherry, putting the juices into a saucepan. Put the cherries on a chopping board and roughly chop them. Add them to the saucepan and bring to the boil. Continue to cook until they are a jammy consistency. Transfer to a bowl to cool.

Put the base of the cake on a serving plate and spread the jam over one side of one sponge.

Place the cream, honey and vanilla in a mixing bowl and whip together. Spread a layer of cream over the jam, reserving the rest to go on top. Put the second sponge on top with the flattest side facing upward.

Pipe or spoon the remaining cream on top. Add the reserved pretty cherries around the edge. Coarsely grate or use a vegetable peeler to make curls of the chocolate and scatter them over the centre. Chill the cake until you are ready to serve.

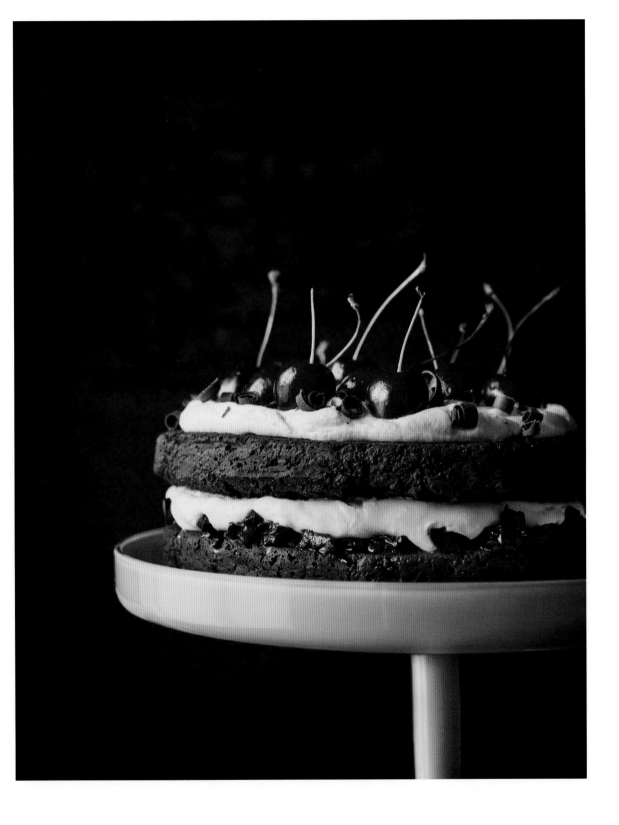

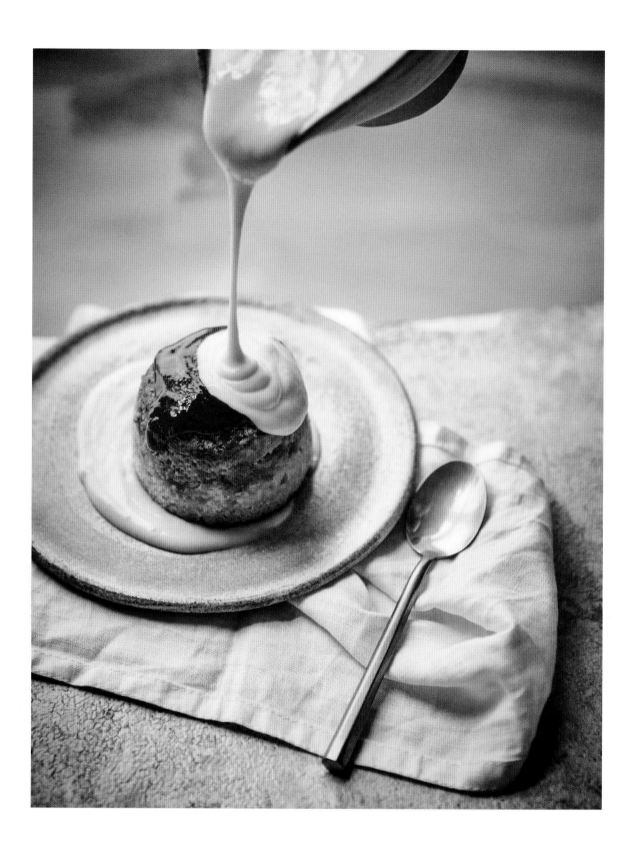

HOT RASPBERRY SPONGE PUDDING

Serves 6

75g (2½oz) butter, softened, plus
    extra for greasing
250g (9oz) fresh or frozen
    raspberries
2 teaspoons vanilla extract
¼ teaspoon almond extract
    (optional)
2 eggs
75g (2½oz) ground almonds
1 tablespoon honey or 2
    tablespoons erythritol
1 teaspoon baking powder

PER SERVING: NET CARBS 6g
FIBRE 4g | PROTEIN 5g
FAT 19g | 223kcal

PER SERVING WITH ERYTHRITOL:
NET CARBS 3g | FIBRE 4g | PROTEIN 5g
FAT 19g | 212kcal

In a typical ready-made sponge pudding there could be up to 63g (2¼oz) of carbs, but ours have just 11g (½oz), so your blood sugar levels won't hit the roof. The butter and almonds in these puddings make them completely delicious but they do push the calories higher, so have them as a special treat, not an everyday occurrence. Individual dariole moulds made from silicone or metal are ideal for this, approximately 6cm (2½ inches) in height and diameter across the top. I have also lined small china coffee cups with wetted and scrunched baking paper and used these too. I use frozen raspberries in winter and fresh in summer to make the jam.

Generously grease 6 approx. 6cm (2½ inch) metal dariole moulds with butter and cut a small circle of baking paper to cover the base of each one. If using silicone moulds there is no need to grease or line them.

Put the raspberries (you can do this from frozen) and 1 teaspoon of the vanilla extract into a saucepan. Bring them to a boil and use a potato masher to mash them to a pulp as they heat and soften. Turn the heat to low and let them simmer gently for 5 minutes, stirring frequently.

Pour the raspberries into a sieve over a bowl and push them through with a spoon until you are left with only the pips to discard. You should be left with a pouring consistency like that of soup. If it is very runny, heat the sauce for a few minutes to reduce and thicken it. Measure out 6 tablespoons of the sauce and keep this to one side as you will need it for serving. Pour the rest into the moulds, divided equally between them.

Heat the oven to 190°C/170°C fan (375°F), Gas Mark 5.

Put the remaining ingredients, including the second teaspoon of vanilla, into a bowl and briefly stir through with a spatula until just combined. If you stir a little too much, the mix may start to separate so don't overdo it (if this happens don't worry as it cooks perfectly).

Spoon the mixture into the moulds and put them into an ovenproof dish. Fill the dish with cold water to come up 3cm (1¼ inches) around the sides of the moulds. Put into the oven for 18–20 minutes or until the sponge is golden brown and feels springy to the touch. Test for doneness with a cocktail stick to make sure it comes out of the centre clean. Carefully remove from the oven and leave them until you are ready to serve: they will sit happily for up to 30 minutes.

When you are ready to serve, briefly heat the extra raspberry sauce in a small pan or in the microwave. Lift the moulds out of the water. If they are still hot, use tongs to do this. Run a knife around the edge of the mould and invert each one on a warm plate with a little of the extra sauce poured over the top. Serve with hot custard, cream or mascarpone.

VANILLA CUSTARD

Serves 6

300ml (10fl oz) full-fat
    unsweetened almond or cows'
    milk
2 egg yolks
seeds scraped from 1 vanilla pod
    or 1½ teaspoons vanilla extract
2 teaspoons honey or 1 heaped
    tablespoon erythritol
15g ½ oz) cornflour

PER SERVING WITH HONEY:
NET CARBS 6g | FIBRE 0g | PROTEIN 3g
FAT 3g | 62kcal

PER SERVING WITH ERYTHRITOL:
NET CARBS 5g | FIBRE 0g | PROTEIN 3g
FAT 3g | 55kcal

To lower the carb count we have used almond milk, as it doesn't contain the milk sugar, lactose. If you can't eat egg, you can use ready-made sugar-free custard powder.

Put the milk, egg yolks, vanilla, honey or erythritol and cornflour into a cold saucepan off the heat. Whisk them together until smooth.

Prepare a piece of baking paper, scrunch it up and dampen it under water, then set aside.

Put the pan over a medium–high heat and keep whisking until the mixture begins to thicken. As soon as this happens, remove the pan from the heat and keep whisking. Cover the surface of the custard with the damp, scrunched baking paper. This will stop the custard from forming a skin. Set aside and leave to cool. You can speed this up by plunging the saucepan into a large bowl of iced water.

COFFEE RICOTTA SHOTS

Serves 6

250g (9oz) ricotta cheese, drained
4 tablespoons cold espresso
2–3 teaspoons honey, to taste, or
  1 heaped teaspoon erythritol, or
  more to taste
2 teaspoons brandy or dark rum
  (optional)
20g (¾oz) dark chocolate (at least
  70% cocoa solids)

PER SERVING WITH HONEY:
NET CARBS 6g | FIBRE 0g | PROTEIN 4g
FAT 6g | 94kcal

PER SERVING WITH ERYTHRITOL:
NET CARBS 4g | FIBRE 0g | PROTEIN 4g
FAT 6g | 87kcal

This is one of my favourite recipes in the book. When Giancarlo was growing up in Tuscany, sweetened ricotta and coffee were eaten as a breakfast or merenda (an afternoon snack), but I now serve this as a dessert. It is perfect served in the old, unmatching, small vintage glasses that I have collected from boot fairs and charity shops over the years.

Whisk the ricotta in a bowl with the coffee, honey or erythritol and the brandy, if using. Taste and adjust the sweetness as necessary, adding more sugar if you wish.

Spoon into small liqueur glasses, taking care not to splash it on the sides of the glass. Use a sharp knife to shave curls of chocolate from a bar and scatter them over the top. Keep them in the refrigerator until you are ready to eat them (up to 1 day). Serve chilled.

FLORENTINES

Makes 12

40g (1½oz) flaked almonds
2 tablespoons double cream
2 teaspoons honey
1 teaspoon vanilla extract
finely grated zest of ½ orange
25g (1oz) butter
100g (3½oz) dark chocolate (at
    least 85% cocoa solids), optional

PER FLORENTINE: NET CARBS 4g
FIBRE 1g | PROTEIN 2g | FAT 8g |
101kcal

Apparently, Florentines don't come from Florence, but were probably invented in France to honour Catherine de Medici who married Henry II of France – and she was from Florence! These nutty, zesty delights can be coated on one side with chocolate or left undressed. Try them instead of a dessert with coffee after a meal.

Heat the oven to 200°C/180°C fan (400°F), Gas Mark 6. Line a baking tray with baking paper.

Spread the almonds over a tray and toast in the oven for 4–5 minutes.

Put the cream, honey, vanilla, zest and butter into a small saucepan and bring to the boil. Let it bubble for a minute and then add the almonds. Stir through and remove from the heat. Leave it to settle and cool for a couple of minutes.

Use a dessertspoon to place 12 mounds, 5cm (2 inches) apart, on the lined baking tray. Flatten them down a little with the back of the spoon and bake the biscuits for 6–8 minutes, or until golden brown. Remove from the oven and use a dinner knife to correct any wonky shapes (unless you like them like that!). Slide the baking paper off the tray and leave the biscuits to cool and set firm.

If you are covering the bases with chocolate, melt the chocolate in a glass basin over a simmering pan of hot water, not allowing it to touch the water. Alternatively, use a microwave. Allow the chocolate to cool to around 26–30°C (79–86°F). You can test this with a thermometer or feel with your finger: it should feel cool.

Use a dinner knife to spread a thin layer of the chocolate on the bases of the biscuits. You can also use the knife to make a criss-cross or wavy design in the setting chocolate. Put the Florentines, chocolate side up, on a cooling rack, or a plate to set and cool.

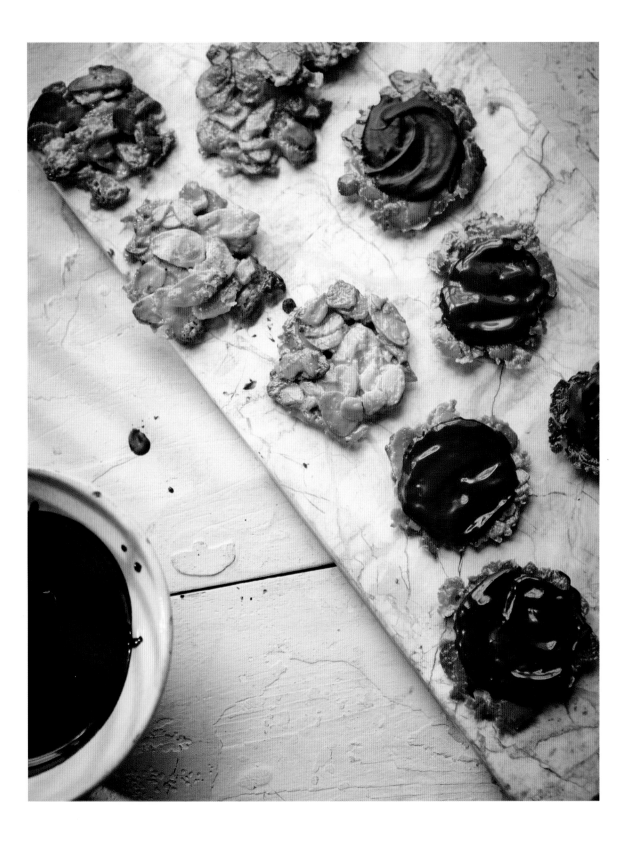

Weekly Meal Plan

Photocopy this plan and fill it in.

	BREAKFAST	LUNCH	DINNER
MONDAY			
TUESDAY			
WEDNESDAY			
THURSDAY			
FRIDAY			
SATURDAY			
SUNDAY			

Further resources

Social Media

Katie Caldesi is on Instagram and X, formerly Twitter, @KatieCaldesi and on Facebook as Katie Caldesi's The Good Kitchen Table. Also see our website www.thegoodkitchentable.com. Our restaurants and cookery schools are at www.caldesi.com

Dr David Unwin is on X, formerly Twitter, @lowcarbGP

Dr Jen Unwin is on Instagram @jen_unwin. For further information on carb addiction see her book *Fork in the Road* (2021) and her website www.forkintheroad.co.uk

Jenny Phillips is on Instagram @jennynutrition and her website is www.inspirednutrition.co.uk

Organizations

The nutritional analysis in this book is only a guide. We use www.cronometer.com. There are so many variables when using nutritional software – ingredients differ around the world and often allowances are not made for fat left at the bottom of a roasting dish or the size of someone else's tablespoon!

Carbs & Cals produce very useful carb and calorie counter books and apps, www.carbsandcals.com

Freestyle Libre makes instant glucose monitoring systems, www.freestylelibre.co.uk

The Public Health Collaboration is a charity dedicated to informing and implementing healthy decisions for better public health, www.phcuk.org.

Diet Doctor has a mass of well researched and evidence-backed information on going low carb and keto, www.dietdoctor.com

Our other books

The Diabetes Weight-loss Cookbook, 2019
The Reverse Your Diabetes Cookbook, 2020
The 30 Minute Diabetes Cookbook, 2021
The Low Carb Weight-loss Cookbook, 2022
The Low Carb Italian Kitchen, 2023

David Unwin's references

1. Unwin D, Delon C, Unwin J, Tobin S, Taylor R. 'What predicts drug-free type 2 diabetes remission? Insights from an 8-year general practice service evaluation of a lower carbohydrate diet with weight loss', in *BMJ Nutrition, Prevention & Health*. 2023:e000544.

2. Rauber F, da Costa Louzada ML, Steele EM, Millett C, Monteiro CA, Levy RB. 'Ultra-Processed Food Consumption and Chronic Non-Communicable Diseases-Related Dietary Nutrient Profile in the UK (2008–2014)', in *Nutrients*. 2018;10(5).

3. Unwin D, Haslam D, Livesey G. 'It is the glycaemic response to, not the carbohydrate content of food that matters in diabetes and obesity: The glycaemic index revisited', in *Journal of Insulin Resistance*. 2016. 2016;1(1).

4. Unwin D, Tobin S. 'A patient request for some "deprescribing"', in BMJ. 2015;351:h4023.

5. Unwin D, Khalid AA, Unwin J, Crocombe D, Delon C, Martyn K, et al. 'Insights from a general practice service evaluation supporting a lower carbohydrate diet in patients with type 2 diabetes mellitus and prediabetes: a secondary analysis of routine clinic data including HbA1c, weight and prescribing over 6 years', in *BMJ Nutrition, Prevention & Health*. 2020:bmjnph-2020-000072.

6. Unwin DJ, Tobin SD, Murray SW, Delon C, Brady AJ. 'Substantial and Sustained Improvements in Blood Pressure, Weight and Lipid Profiles from a Carbohydrate Restricted Diet: An Observational Study of Insulin Resistant Patients in Primary Care', in *International Journal of Environmental Research and Public Health*. 2019;16(15):2680.

7. Insights from a general practice service evaluation supporting a lower carbohydrate diet in patients with type 2 diabetes mellitus and prediabetes: Unwin, D., et al., BMJ Nutrition, Prevention & Health, 2020: p. bmjnph-2020-000071.

8. What predicts drug-free type 2 diabetes remission? Insights from an 8-year general practice service evaluation of a carbohydrate diet. Unwin D. Taylor R. et al. BMJ Nutrition.

9. Cunnane SC, Courchesne-Loyer A, St-Pierre V, Vandenberghe C, Pierotti T, Fortier M, et al. 'Can ketones compensate for deteriorating brain glucose uptake during aging? Implications for the risk and treatment of Alzheimer's disease.', in *Annals of the New York Academy of Sciences*. 2016;1367(1):12-20.

Additional Picture Credits

Index

A huge thank you to

Our publisher Joanna Copestick

Everyone who helped me with this book including our boys Giorgio and Flavio, Stefano Borella, the Soin family and Ann Hudson

Jonathan Hayden, our literary agent

Isabel Jessop, editor, for bringing the project together so calmly

Maja Smend for the stunning photography

Lizzie Harris for the beautiful food styling

Sarah Birks for the prop styling

Paul Palmer-Edwards for the design of the book

Katherine Hockley for the production

Nadine Radford, KC, for additional proofreading

Giancarlo, Jenny and I were delighted to work with Dr David Unwin and Dr Jen Unwin on this project. Their knowledge, experience and help were invaluable. We wish it to be known that they have received no fee for their participation in this book. Instead, we made a donation to the Public Health Collaboration to further their work spreading the real food message.